Breakthrough Health

Ted and Sharon Broer

Breakthrough Health
Ted Broer

Published by B&A Publications
P.O.Box 125
Auburndale, Florida 33823

Library of Congress cataloging-in-Publication data
ISBN: 978-1-59755-360-5

This book is not intended to take the place of any medical advice and or treatment from
your personal physician. Readers are advised to consult their own doctor or other
qualified health professionals regarding the treatment of their medical problems. Neither
the publisher, Healthmasters nor the author takes any responsibility for any possible
consequences from any treatment, action or application of medicine, supplement, herb or
preparation to any person reading or following the information in this book. Do not stop
taking any medication issued by prescription without first consulting with your medical
doctor or health care provider.

Printed in the United States of America

DEDICATION

Sharon and I have been married for thirty years. During that time, we have done our best to keep our customers, readers, and listeners updated on the latest health, nutrition, and supplement news and development as possible.

Sharon's mother, Shirley Bennett, has been with us the whole journey, offering continual support. She has not only supported our efforts, but has listened to us for her nutritional needs and uses our suggested products.

Shirley, at the time of this publication, was on a motor home trip in the western part of the United States, traveling alone, to fulfill a dream which began with her deceased husband as of a year ago. In the final weeks prior to the publication of our book, Shirley interrupted her trip to help us edit this manuscript.

Being 78 years old, she has excellent mental acuity, is physically active (playing golf several times a week), and is on zero medications. She is a true testament to the benefits of eating right, of exercising and of taking of high quality supplements.

Sharon and I want to dedicate this book to "Mom," Shirley Bennett, without whom this book would not have been possible.

TABLE OF CONTENTS

▌ Bad, Bad Medicine

I still shake my head in disbelief when I think of this: U.S. government agencies continue to claim that vitamins (yes, vitamins!) are hazardous to our health, while they ignore the lawsuits, the negative press, the industry reports and statistics that prove how unsafe 'approved' pharmaceuticals really are. How is this allowed to continue?

Fortunately, a dedicated group of researchers compiled and analyzed all of the published information available that addresses the deaths and injuries caused by prescriptions. The researchers concluded that the current system causes more harm than it does good. Here are the details of that finding:

Each year:

- 2.2 million have in-hospital adverse reactions to prescribed drugs;
- 20 million antibiotics are prescribed unnecessarily for viral infections;
- 7.5 million unnecessary medical and surgical procedures are performed;
- 8.9 million people are unnecessarily hospitalized.

As dramatic as that appears, here's the stat that really stopped me in my tracks.

Nearly 784,000 deaths are caused by conventional medicine each year, making our medical system the leading cause of death in America. That's more than heart disease and more than cancer!

Do our medical professionals know these stats? Some do and hopefully they are going against the status quo to do what they can to help turn these numbers around.

Iatrogenic is a term used when a patient dies as a direct result of treatments by a physician, whether it is from misdiagnosis of the ailment or from adverse drug reactions used to treat the illness. (drug reactions are the most common cause).

Any invasive, unnecessary medical procedure must be considered as part of the larger iatrogenic picture. The figures on unnecessary events represent a one-year time span for 16.4 million people who suddenly find themselves at the mercy of a dangerous health care system. A hospital visit, no matter the length, could result in any of the following potentially fatal consequences:

- A 2.1% chance (affecting 186,000) of a serious adverse drug reaction. Incidence of adverse drug reactions in hospitalized patients: a meta-analysis of prospective studies. JAMA
- A 5-6% chance (affecting 489,500) of acquiring a nosocomial infection. Nosocomial Infection Update. Emerging Infectious Diseases journal — CDC
- A 4 -36% chance (affecting 1.78 million) of having an iatrogenic injury (medical error and adverse drug reactions). Error in Medicine, JAMA
- A 17% chance (affecting 1.3 million) of a procedure error. Medication errors in hospitalized cardiovascular patients. JAMA Intern Medicine

Over the course of 10 years, 7.8 million iatrogenic deaths could occur. That's more casualties than what was suffered in every war in U.S. history.

Is American Medicine Working?

In 2010, public and private healthcare spending totaled $2.6 trillion, representing 17.9% of the U.S. economy, the same proportion as in 2009, according to a government report released in 2012.

Considering this enormous expenditure, we should have the best medicine in the world. We should be preventing and reversing disease, and doing minimal harm. We're a long way from that scenario.

Healthcare spending rose 3.8% in 2009, the smallest rise in the 51 years that the federal Centers for Medicare & Medicaid Services has been tracking the data. It rose 3.9% in 2010. The increase represents the second-lowest rate on record as consumers avoided going to the doctor, taking expensive prescription drugs and undergoing costly elective procedures.

It is widely acknowledged that within the U.S. there is no clear link between higher spending on health care and longer life, less disability or better quality of life. A 2003 study published in Annals of Internal Medicine found that Medicare patients who lived in areas with higher health care spending did not get better results. In some cases, more spending even appears to equal poorer health. A 2004 study in Health Affairs found that there was actually worse care in states with higher Medicare spending.

And instead of minimizing various disease-causing factors, we cause more illness through medical technology, diagnostic testing, overuse of medical and surgical procedures, and overuse of pharmaceutical drugs. The huge disservice of this therapeutic strategy is the result of little effort or money being spent on preventing disease.

UNDER-REPORTING
OF IATROGENIC EVENTS

Less than 20% of iatrogenic acts are ever reported, which may be the second biggest roadblock to fully reforming medicine from the curriculum in medical schools to protecting patients from excessive medical intervention. The first, and perhaps most important, are the powerful pharmaceutical and medical technology companies, along with other powerful groups with enormous vested interests in the business of medicine. They fund medical research, support medical schools and hospitals, and advertise in medical journals. With deep pockets, they entice scientists and academics to support their efforts. Such funding can sway the balance of opinion from professional caution to uncritical acceptance of new therapies and drugs. You have only to look at the people who make up the hospital, medical, and government health advisory boards to see conflicts of interest.

Consider the 2003 study that found that nearly half of medical school faculties who serve on institutional review boards (IRB) to advise on clinical trial research also serve as consultants to the pharmaceutical industry. And the public is mostly unaware of these interlocking interests.

MEDICAL ETHICS AND CONFLICT
OF INTEREST IN SCIENTIFIC MEDICINE

When Jonathan Quick was director of essential drugs and medicines policy for the World Health Organization (WHO), he wrote: "If clinical trials become a commercial venture in which self-interest overrules public interest and desire overrules science, then the social contract which allows research on human subjects in return for medical advances is broken."

Dr. Marcia Angell, a former editor of the New England Journal of Medicine, agreed with him in her editorial entitled " Is Academic Medicine for Sale?"

"When the boundaries between industry and academic medicine become as blurred as they are now, the business goals of industry influence the mission of medical schools in multiple ways." According to an ABC news report, pharmaceutical companies spend over $2 billion a year on over 314,000 events attended by doctors.

The ABC news report also noted that a survey of clinical trials revealed that when a drug company funds a study, there is a 90% chance that the drug will be perceived as effective, whereas, a non-drug-company-funded study will show favorable results only 50% of the time. It appears that money can't buy what you love, but it can buy any "scientific" result desired.

PUBLIC SUGGESTIONS ON IATROGENESIS

In a Reuters Health telephone survey, 1,207 adults ranked the effectiveness of the following measures in reducing preventable medical errors that result in serious harm. (Following each measure is the percentage of respondents who ranked the measure as "very effective.")

- Giving doctors more time to spend with patients (78%)
- Requiring hospitals to develop systems to avoid medical errors (74%)
- Better training of health professionals (73%)
- Using only doctors specially trained in intensive care medicine on intensive care units (73%)
- Requiring hospitals to report all serious medical errors to a state agency (71%)
- Increasing the number of hospital nurses (69%)
- Reducing the work hours of doctors in training to avoid fatigue (66%)
- Encouraging hospitals to voluntarily report serious medical errors to a state agency (62%).

DRUG IATROGENESIS

Modern scientific medicine relies on treatment largely by use of prescription drugs. Though the public had accepted the prevailing 'germ theory' – that infectious organisms were the cause of illness — establishing a 'cure' for these infections wasn't as easy as science had hoped. And while chemical drugs were incredibly effective, their side effects were anything but encouraging. Even when dispensed properly, Lazarou discovered that the drugs could still have fatal side effects. Add to that the possibly of human error, and a situation dramatically worsened.

Medicating Our Feelings

Patients seeking freedom from anxiety, worry, depression and stress, end up succumbing to the carefully worded seduction of prescription drug ads on television and in magazines. And, then the side effects of antidepressant medication sets in. Something these patients may be used to having happen. After all, a whole generation of antidepressant users has been created from young people growing up on Ritalin; A generation who prefers to modify their emotions rather than learn to deal with their feelings.

Of course, the downside is that as adults, their coping mechanism is found in the shape of a beer bottle or more pills.

Television Diagnosis

Contrary to what Big Pharma tells you, the U.S. pharmaceutical industry spends almost twice as much on promotion as it does on research and development. And the bulk of that money is spent on direct advertising of prescription drugs to women.

Currently, Big Pharma spends $4.2 billion on advertising, up to 19 times more than it spends on researching and developing new drugs.

A separate study found " that people mistakenly believe that the FDA reviews all ads before they are released and allows only the safest and most effective drugs to be promoted directly to the public." A advertising industry insider noted, "If the general public knew how every word, phrase, positioning and other aspects of these ads are scrutinized, labored over and evaluated for maximum profit to the company, they would all realize that patient well-being has little to do with the process."

How Do We Know Drugs Are Safe?

The testing of new drugs is taken for granted and trusted by the public. Here's the problem with that: Typically, drugs are tested on healthy individuals not taking any other medication which could mar a finding. Once that drug test is over and the drug is deemed safe, then another phase of testing comes into play — the post approval phase. Here, the side effects are documented after the drug has hit the streets. As an example of this phase, a report from the federal government's General Accounting Office "found that of the 198 drugs approved by the FDA between 1976 and 1985 . . . 102 (more than half) had serious post-approval risks . . . the serious post-approval risks (included) heart failure, myocardial infarction, anaphylaxis, respiratory depression and arrest, seizures, kidney and liver failure, severe blood disorders, birth defects and fetal toxicity, and blindness."

Recently, the NBC show "Dateline" investigated if our doctors are moonlighting as drug company representatives. After a year-long investigation, Dateline reported that because doctors can legally prescribe any drug to any patient for any condition, drug companies heavily promote "off label." Off-label indicates frequently inappropriate and untested uses of any given medications — despite being approved only for the specific indications for which they have been tested.

To date, the leading causes of adverse drug reactions are antibiotics (17%), cardiovascular drugs (17%), chemotherapy (15%), and analgesics and anti-inflammatory agents (15%).

2 | Medical and Surgical Procedures

Despite its commonplace and a patient's perception that the surgery is safe and necessary, even the most routine medical and surgical procedure has an inherent risk associated with it. It's no wonder that allopathic medicine itself is a leading cause of death.

One reason is the perception that allopathic medicine is all about 'health care'. That couldn't be further from the truth. Allopathic medicine is about profit-driven 'disease care'. And while the HCUP figures are helpful, the system for calculating annual mortality statistics for all U.S. hospital discharges is flawed. A HCUP email revealed that the mortality rates for each procedure indicated only that the patient undergoing that procedure died either from the procedure or from some other cause. As a result, it was impossible to tell how many people die from a specific procedure. And the figures for mortalities categorized "poisoning & toxic effects of drugs" and "complications of treatment" are available, they don't include the mortality figures registered in these categories: No codes exist for things like adverse drug side effects, surgical mishaps, or other types of medical error. This is why, currently, it's impossible to differentiate the true mortality rates tied to medical error.

An Honest Assessment of U.S. Health Care

In 1978, the U.S. Office of Technology Assessment (OTA) made the claim that "only 10-20% of all procedures currently used in medical practice have been shown to be efficacious by controlled trial."

Before disbanding in 1995, the OTA compared medical technology in eight countries (Australia , Canada, France, Germany, the Netherlands, Sweden, the UK, and the U.S.) and noted that not much had changed: few medical procedures in the U.S. have been subjected to clinical trial. It also reported that U.S. infant mortality was high and life expectancy low compared to other developed countries.

Although nearly 20 years old, much of what was written in the OTA report still holds true today. The report points to the high cost of American medicine on the medical free-enterprise system and failure to create a national health care policy. It also attributes the government's failure to control health care costs to market incentives and profit motives inherent in the current financing and organization of health care, which includes such interests as private health insurers, hospital systems, physicians, and the drug and medical-device industries.

SURGICAL ERRORS FINALLY REPORTED

An October 2004 JAMA study from the AHRQ addressed surgical injuries and "documented 32,000 mostly surgery related deaths costing $9 billion and accounting for 2.4 million extra days in the hospital in 2000." The report further comments that, "The findings greatly underestimate the problem, since many other complications happen that are not listed in hospital administrative data."

Data from 20% of the nation's hospitals were analyzed for 18 different surgical complications, including postoperative infections, foreign objects left in wounds, surgical wounds reopening, and post-operative bleeding. Said AHRQ director Carolyn M. Clancy, MD, "This study gives us the first direct evidence that medical injuries pose a real threat to the American public and increase the costs of health care."

According to the study's authors, "The message here is that medical injuries can have a devastating impact on the health care system. We need more research to identify why these injuries occur and find ways to prevent them from happening."

The study authors also said that improved medical practices, including an emphasis on better hand washing, might help reduce morbidity and mortality rates. In an accompanying JAMA editorial, prominent health care quality expert Dr. Saul Weingart then wrote, "Given their staggering magnitude, these estimates are clearly sobering."

UNNECESSARY X-RAYS

In the early days of x-ray discovery, no one had any idea of the effects of long-term exposure to ionizing radiation. Monthly fluoroscopic exams at the doctor's office (and at most shoe stores) were quite the routine in the 1950's.

Back then, it was common to x-ray pregnant women to measure their pelvises and make a diagnosis of twins. Once a study of 700,000 children born between 1947 and 1964 confirmed that cancer mortality was 40% higher among children whose mothers had been x-rayed, the practice stopped.

These days, coronary angiography is an invasive surgical procedure that involves snaking a tube through a blood vessel in the groin up to the heart. To obtain useful information, X-rays are taken almost continuously, with minimum dosages ranging from 460 to 1,580 mrem. The minimum radiation from a routine chest x-ray is 2 mrem. X-ray radiation accumulates in the body, and ionizing radiation used in X-ray procedures has been shown to cause gene mutation. The health impact of this high level of radiation is unknown, and often obscured in statistical jargon such as, "The risk for lifetime fatal cancer due to radiation exposure is estimated to be 4 in one million per 1,000 mrem," states the Journal of the National Cancer Institute.

Before he died in 2007, Dr. John Gofman was the nation's leading medical physicist, having studied the effects of radiation on human health for 45 years. In addition to working on the Manhattan Project, he discovered uranium-233, and was the first person to isolate plutonium. He also believed that medical technology — x-rays, CT scans, and mammography and fluoroscopy devices — are contributing factors to 75% of new cancers. In his 700-page report, "Radiation from Medical Procedures in the Pathogenesis of Cancer and Ischemic Heart Disease: Dose-Response Studies with Physicians per 100,000 Population," he shows that as the number of physicians increases in a geographical area along with an increase in the number of x-ray diagnostic tests performed, the rate of cancer and ischemic heart disease also increases. He has also predicted that ionizing radiation will be responsible for 100 million premature deaths over the next decade.

In his book, "Preventing Breast Cancer," Dr. Gofman noted that breast cancer is the leading cause of death among American women between the ages of 44 and 55. Because breast tissue is highly sensitive to radiation, mammograms, he said, past exposure to ionizing radiation — primarily medical x-rays — is responsible for about 75 percent of the breast-cancer problem in the United States. The good news is that since the radiation dosage given today by medical procedures can be significantly reduced without interfering with a single useful procedure, numerous future cases of breast-cancer can be prevented.

UNNECESSARY HOSPITALIZATION

Nearly 9 million people were hospitalized unnecessarily in 2001, according to the Agency for Healthcare Research and Quality. In a study of inappropriate hospitalization, two doctors reviewed 1,132 medical records and concluded that 23% of all admissions were inappropriate and another 17% could have been handled in outpatient clinics. Overall, 34 percent of all hospital days were deemed inappropriate and could have been avoided. The rate of inappropriate hospital admissions in 1990 was 23.5%. In 1999, the American Journal of Public Health also reported an inappropriate admissions rate of 24%. The Healthcare Cost and Utilization Project (Healthcare Research and Quality) database indicated that of the 37,187,641 total number of patient discharges from U.S. hospitals in 2001, nearly nine million people were potential iatrogenic episodes.

3 | Women's Experience In Medicine

Jean-Martin Charcot was a French neurologist and professor of anatomical pathology. He is known as "the founder of modern neurology" (1825-1893) was the most celebrated doctor of his time and an expert in hysteria, diagnosing an average of 10 hysterical women each day, transforming them into "iatrogenic monsters" and turning simple "neurosis" into hysteria. Hysteria is derived from the Latin "hystera" meaning uterus. According to Dr. Adriane Fugh-Berman — an Associate Professor in the Department of Pharmacology and Physiology and in the Department of Family Medicine at Georgetown University Medical Center — U.S. medicine has a tradition of excessive medical and surgical interventions on women. Only 100 years ago, male doctors believed that female psychological imbalance originated in the uterus. When surgery to remove the uterus was perfected, it became the "cure" for mental instability, effecting a physical and psychological castration. Fugh-Berman notes that U.S. doctors eventually disabused themselves of that notion but have continued to treat women very differently than they treat men. She cites the following statistics:

- Thousands of prophylactic mastectomies are performed annually.
- One-third of U.S. women have had a hysterectomy prior to menopause.
- Women are prescribed drugs more frequently than are men.
- Women are given potent drugs for disease prevention, which results in disease substitution due to side effects.
- Fetal monitoring is unsupported by studies and not recommended by the CDC. It confines women to a hospital bed and may result in a higher incidence of cesarean section.
- Normal processes such as menopause and childbirth have been heavily "medicalized."

- Synthetic hormone replacement therapy (HRT) does not prevent heart disease or dementia, but does increase the risk of breast cancer, heart disease, stroke, and gall bladder attack.

As reported by JAMA, nearly one-third of postmenopausal women use HRT. This number is important in light of the much publicized Women's Health Initiative Study, which was halted before its completion because of a higher death rate in the synthetic estrogen-progestin (HRT) group.

Cesarean Section

In 1983, cesarean sections were the nation's most common obstetric-gynecologic (OB/GYN) surgical procedure. The second most common procedure was Hysterectomies, followed by diagnostic dilation and curettage of the uterus (632,000). That same year OB/GYN procedures represented 23% of all surgery completed in the U.S. By 2001, C-sections are still the most common OB/GYN surgical procedure, having risen to 960,000 from 673,000 just seven years later. That's 24 percent of the approximately four million births that year. In the Netherlands, only 8% of births are delivered by cesarean. One might conclude that 640,000 unnecessary C-sections — with three to four times higher mortality and 20 times greater morbidity than vaginal delivery — are performed annually in the U.S.

NEVER ENOUGH STUDIES

Whether to reveal the dangers of DDT and other pesticides before instituting a ban or disputing the connection between tobacco and lung cancer, when it served their purpose to do so, scientists have long claimed there simply wasn't enough research to tell us what we now know. (What we've always known.) No surprise there. Even the American Medical Association (AMA) went as far as to not endorse the Surgeon General's 1964 report when he condemned smoking. The AMA's reason? It needed more research. Really! What they were waiting for — and ultimately received – was nine years' worth of payments which totaled $18 million from — you guessed it — a consortium of tobacco companies. And in exchange, the AMA said nothing about the dangers of smoking for almost a decade.

4 | The First Itrogenic Study

Dr. Lucian Leape, a health policy analyst whose research has spotlighted patient safety and quality of care, published the "Harvard Medical Practice Study" in 1991, which found a 4 percent iatrogenic injury rate for patients, with a 14 percent fatality rate in 1984 in New York State. Using the 98,609 patients injured and the 14 percent fatality rate, he estimated that in the entire U.S., 180,000 people die each year partly as a result of iatrogenic injury.

People have questioned his choice of using the much lower figure of 4% injury for his analysis, suggesting that using the average of the rates found in the three studies he cites (36%, 20%, and 4%) would have produced a 20 percent medical error rate or 1,189,576 deaths.

Leape acknowledged that the literature on medical errors is sparse and represents only the tip of the iceberg, noting that when errors are specifically sought out, reported rates are "distressingly high." He cited several autopsy studies with rates as high as 35-40% of missed diagnoses causing death. He also noted that an intensive care unit reported an average of 1.7 errors per day per patient, and 29% of those errors were potentially serious or fatal.

Leape calculated the error rate in the intensive care unit study. First, he found that each patient had an average of 178 "activities" (staff/procedure/medical interactions) a day, of which 1.7 were errors, which means a 1 percent failure rate. This may not seem like much, but Leape cited industry standards showing that in aviation, a 0.1% failure rate would mean two unsafe plane landings per day at Chicago's O'Hare International Airport; in the US Postal Service, a 0.1 percent failure rate would mean 16,000 pieces of mail lost every hour; and in the banking industry, a 0.1 percent failure rate would mean 32,000 bank checks deducted from the wrong bank account.

In trying to determine why there are so many medical errors, Leape acknowledged the lack of reporting of medical errors. He said that the problem of medical errors is largely unrecognized and growing because doctors and nurses are "unequipped to deal with human error due to the culture of medical training and practice."

Doctors are taught that mistakes are unacceptable. Medical mistakes are therefore viewed as a failure of character and any error equals negligence. No one is taught what to do when medical errors do occur. Leape cites McIntyre and Popper, who said the "infallibility model" of medicine leads to intellectual dishonesty with a need to cover up mistakes rather than admit them. There are no Grand Rounds on medical errors, no sharing of failures among doctors, and no one to support them emotionally when their error harms a patient.

Leape hoped his paper would encourage medical practitioners "to fundamentally change the way they think about errors and why they occur." Unfortunately, more than two decades later, the problem still persists.

In 1995, JAMA noted, "Over a million patients are injured in U.S. hospitals each year and approximately 280,000 die annually as a result of these injuries. Therefore, the iatrogenic death rate dwarfs the annual automobile accident mortality rate of 45,000 and accounts for more deaths than all other accidents combined."

In 1997 Leape revealed that more than 100 million Americans have been affected directly or indirectly by a medical mistake. Forty-two percent were affected directly and 84 percent personally knew of someone who had experienced a medical mistake. He also noted that medical errors in inpatient hospital settings nationwide could be as high as 3 million and could cost as much as $200 billion.

ONLY A FRACTION OF MEDICAL ERRORS ARE REPORTED

In 1994, Leape acknowledged that a huge majority of medical errors were not being reported. A study conducted in a pair of UK obstetrical units found that only about one-quarter of adverse incidents were ever reported. The reasoning? To either protect staff, preserve reputations, or avoid reprisals, including lawsuits. An analysis by H.L. Wald and Kaveh Shojania, researchers specializing in medical error, patient safety and quality improvement, found that only 1.5% of all adverse events result in an incident report, and only 6% of adverse drug events are ever identified properly. The authors learned that the American College of Surgeons estimates that surgical incident reports routinely captures just 5-30% of adverse events. The Journal of Evaluation in Clinical Practice reported that in one, only 20% of surgical complications resulted in discussion at morbidity and mortality rounds. From these studies, it appears that all the statistics gathered on medical errors may substantially underestimate the number of adverse drug and medical therapy incidents.

An April 2000 Psychiatric Times article examined the reluctance to report medical errors. The authors found that the public is fearful of suffering a fatal medical error, and doctors are afraid they will be sued if they report one. So who, then, is actually reporting the medical errors? Typically it's the patient or the patients surviving family. If no one notices the error, it is never reported. Janet Heinrich, an associate director at the U.S. General Accounting Office responsible for health financing and public health issues, testified before a House subcommittee hearing on medical errors that "the full magnitude of their threat to the American public is unknown" and "gathering valid and useful information about adverse events is extremely difficult." She stated in frank language, that the fear of being blamed, and the potential for legal liability, played key roles in the under reporting of errors. The Psychiatric Times also noted that the AMA strongly opposes mandatory reporting of medical errors. That leaves nurses — but a survey of their attitudes toward reporting medical errors (Psychiatric Times, April 2000) revealed they failed to report out of fear of retaliation.

According to *Journal of Applied Communication Research*, standard medical pharmacology texts reveal that relatively few doctors ever report adverse drug reactions to the FDA, for reasons ranging from from not knowing such a reporting system exists, to fear of being sued. Yet the public depends on this tremendously flawed system of voluntary reporting by doctors to know whether a drug or a medical intervention is actually harmful.

Pharmacology texts also will tell doctors how hard it is to discern drug side effects from disease symptoms: Treatment failure is most often attributed to the disease and not the drug or doctor. Even at their training stage, doctors are forewarned, "Probably nowhere else in professional life are mistakes so easily hidden, even from ourselves." Perhaps that's why — as incredible as it sounds — only 1 in 20 side effects is actually reported to either hospital administrators or the FDA.

If hospitals admitted to the actual number of errors for which they were responsible (which we know is about 20 times what is actually reported), they would constantly be under intense scrutiny. Jerry Phillips, former associate director of the FDA's Office of Post Marketing Drug Risk Assessment, confirmed this number to JAMA. "In the broader area of adverse drug reaction data, the 250,000 reports received annually probably represent only 5 percent of the actual reactions that occur." Dr. Jay Cohen, who has extensively researched adverse drug reactions, notes that because only 5 percent of adverse drug reactions are reported, there are, in fact, five million medication reactions each year.

The results of another 2003 survey is equally distressing because there seems to be no improvement in error reporting, even with all the attention given to the subject. Dr. Dorothea Wild surveyed medical residents at a community hospital in Connecticut and she was astonished at what she discovered: only half the medical residents were aware that the hospital had a medical error-reporting system, and nearly no one ever used it. "This does not bode well for the future," she said. "If doctors don't learn error reporting in their training, they'll never use it." Wild adds that error reporting is the first step in locating the gaps in the medical system and fixing them. "But not even that first step has been taken to date."

MEDICATION ERRORS

A survey of a 1992 national pharmacy database found a total of 429,827 medication errors from 1,081 hospitals.

According to a 2002 survey by the Aiser Family Foundation, Harvard School of Public Health, medication mistakes occurred in 5.22 percent of patients admitted to these hospitals each year. The authors concluded that annually, at least 90,895 patients were harmed by medication errors in the U.S., nationwide.

Another 2002 study showed that 20 percent of hospital medications for patients had dosage errors, and that nearly 40 percent of these errors were considered potentially harmful to the patient. Statistically, in a typical 300-patient hospital, the number of errors per day was 40.

Problems involving patients' medications were even higher the following year. The error rate intercepted by pharmacists in this study was 24 percent, making the potential minimum number of patients harmed by prescription drugs 417,908.

Recent Adverse Drug Reactions:

Is the number of adverse drug reactions rising? A study published in 2003 JAMA that compares events between 1994 and 2003 says that may be what's happening. In 2003, 400 patients were followed after discharge from a tertiary care hospital setting (requiring highly specialized skills, technology, or support services). Seventy-six patients (19 percent) had adverse events. Adverse drug events were the most common, at 66 percent of all events. The next most common event was procedure-related injuries, at 17 percent.

A *New England Journal of Medicine* study says that one out of four patients suffered observable side effects from the more than 3.34 billion prescription drugs filled in 2002. One of the doctors who produced the study was interviewed by Reuters and commented, "With these 10-minute appointments, it's hard for the doctor to get into whether the symptoms are bothering the patients."

William Tierney, of the Indiana School of Medicine, said this: "They found that adverse drug events were fairly frequent and usually mild, although potentially serious, and preventable events were more frequent than any patient or clinician would like or should be willing to accept."

"Given the increasing number of powerful drugs available to care for the aging population, the problem will only get worse."

It's been reported that the drugs with the worst record of side effects were selective serotonin reuptake inhibitors (SSRIs), nonsteroidal anti-inflammatory drugs (NSAIDs), and calcium-channel blockers. Reuters also reported that prior research has suggested that nearly 5 percent of hospital admissions (over 1 million per year) are the result of drug side effects. But most of the cases are not documented as such. The study found that one of the reasons for this failure is that in nearly two-thirds of the cases, doctors could not diagnose drug side effects or the side effects persisted because the doctor failed to heed the warning signs.

5 | Specific Drug Itrogenic: Antibiotics

William Agger, MD, director of microbiology and chief of infectious disease at Gundersen Lutheran Medical Center in La Crosse, WI, believes Americans are overusing antibiotics and that overuse results in food-borne infections resistant to antibiotics.

Though Salmonella is found in 20 percent of ground meat, the constant exposure of cattle to antibiotics has made 84 percent of salmonella strains resistant to at least one anti-salmonella antibiotic. Diseased animal food accounts for 80 percent of salmonellosis in humans, or 1.4 million cases per year. The conventional approach to countering this epidemic is to radiate food to try to kill all organisms while continuing to use the antibiotics that created the problem in the first place. Approximately 20 percent of chickens are contaminated with Campylobacter jejuni, an organism that causes 2.4 million cases of illness annually. Fifty-four percent of these organisms are resistant to at least one anti-campylobacter antimicrobial agent.

Denmark banned growth-promoting antibiotics beginning in 1999, which cut their use by more than half within a year, from 453,200 to 195,800 pounds. A report from Scandinavia found that removing antibiotic growth promoters had no or minimal effect on food production costs. Agger warns that the current crowded, unsanitary methods of animal farming in the US support constant stress and infection, and are geared toward high antibiotic use.

In the U.S., over 3 million pounds of antibiotics are used every year on humans. With a population of 284 million Americans, this amount is enough to give every man, woman, and child 10 teaspoons of pure antibiotics per year.

Agger says that exposure to a steady stream of antibiotics has altered pathogens such as Streptococcus pneumoniae, Staplococcus aureus, and entercocci, to name a few.

Almost half of patients with upper respiratory tract infections in the U.S. still receive antibiotics from their doctor, says the Wisconsin Medical Journal. According to the CDC, 90 percent of upper respiratory infections are viral and should not be treated with antibiotics. In Germany, the prevalence of systemic antibiotic use in children aged 0-6 years was 42.9%, reports JAMA Pediatrics.

According to the Journal: Pharmacoepidemiol Drug Safety, data obtained from nine U.S. health insurers on antibiotic use in 25,000 children from 1996 to 2000, found that rates of antibiotic use decreased. Antibiotic use in children aged three months to under 3 years decreased 24%, from 2.46 to 1.89 antibiotic prescriptions per patient per year. For children aged 3 to under 6 years, there was a 25% reduction from 1.47 to 1.09 antibiotic prescriptions per patient per year. And for children aged 6 to under 18 years, there was a 16 percent reduction from 0.85 to 0.69 antibiotic prescriptions per patient per year. Despite these reductions, the data indicate that on average every child in America receives 1.22 antibiotic prescriptions annually.

Group A beta-hemolytic streptococci is the only common cause of sore throat that requires antibiotics, with penicillin and erythromycin the only recommended treatment. Ninety percent of sore-throat cases, however, are viral. Antibiotics were used in 73% of the estimated 6.7 million adult annual visits for sore throat in the US between 1989 and 1999.

A report in Pediatrics magazine noted that patients treated with antibiotics were prescribed non-recommended broad-spectrum antibiotics in 68 percent of visits. This period saw a significant increase in the use of newer, more expensive broad-spectrum antibiotics and a decrease in use of the recommended antibiotics penicillin and erythromycin. Antibiotics being prescribed in 73 percent of sore-throat cases instead of the recommended 10 percent resulted in a total of 4.2 million unnecessary antibiotic prescriptions written between 1989 to 1999.

The Problem with Antibiotics:

It has been 10 years now since the Center for Disease Control re-launched "Get Smart: Know When Antibiotics Work." campaign. The goal of the $1.6 million campaign is to educate patients about the overuse and inappropriate use of antibiotics.

Most healthcare professionals involved with alternative medicine are already well-versed in the dangers of antibiotic overuse. It's a step in the right direction that our government is finally paying attention to an iatrogenic epidemic that has already cost billions of dollars and thousands of lives.

When are antibiotics needed? Only, If you or your child is diagnosed with strep throat, which is caused by bacteria. Strep throat cannot be diagnosed by looking in the throat – a lab test must also be done. Antibiotics are prescribed for strep throat for the purpose of preventing rheumatic fever. If the test result shows strep throat, the infected patient should stay home from work, school, or day care until 24 hours after starting an antibiotic.

Conversely, says the CDC, 90 percent of upper respiratory infections, including children's ear infections, are viral and that antibiotics do not treat viral infection. Each time you or your child takes an antibiotic, the bacteria that normally live in your body (on the skin, in the intestine, in the mouth and nose, etc.) are more likely to become resistant to antibiotics. Common antibiotics cannot kill infections caused by these resistant germs.

Each year about 50 million prescriptions for antibiotics are written in physicians' offices. About 40 percent of those are inappropriate and their misuse can lead to the development of deadly strains of bacteria that are resistant to drugs. These are the same strains of bacteria that and cause more than 88,000 deaths as a result of hospital-acquired infections.

According to 'Get Smart' head, Dr. Richard Besser, says, the program teaches patients and the general public that antibiotics are precious resources that must be used correctly if we want to have them around when we need them. Hopefully, as a result of this campaign, patients will feel more comfortable asking their doctors for the best care for their illnesses, rather than asking for antibiotics."

Drug Companies Fined

Every once in a great while, the FDA slaps the wrist of a drug manufacturer — HARD — when its abuses are just too blatant to ignore or its behavior is too reprehensible to be swept under the carpet by donations to charities and a flurry of press releases. A few years back Schering-Plough Corp., (Levitra, Vytorin, Nasonex and NuvaRing) was indicted on fraud charges and forced to pay a $500 million dollar fine to the U.S. Treasury for quality-control issues around its albuterol inhaler. Allegedly the company distributed the inhalers even though it knew the units were missing the active ingredient.

The FDA tabulated infractions involving 125 products, or 90% of the drugs made by Schering-Plough since 1998. In addition to the fine, Schering was ordered to halt production on 73 of its drugs — or pay another $175 million fine.

Did this industry hear this warning shot? You bet it did, especially since a federal appeals court ruled in 1999 that the FDA could seize the profits of companies that violated "good manufacturing practices."

But Big Pharma needed to be reminded (again) who was in charge. Last year, five pharmaceutical companies agreed to pay nearly $5.5 billion to resolve U.S. Department of Justice allegations of fraudulent marketing practices, including the promotion of medicines for uses that were not approved by the Food and Drug Administration.

For all your nutritional needs **800-726-1834** or **863 967-8484** · **www.Healthmasters.com**   **17**

6 | Unnecessary Surgical Procedures

In 1974, 2.4 million unnecessary surgeries were performed, resulting in 11,900 deaths at a cost of $3.9 billion (73,74). In 2001, 7.5 million unnecessary surgical procedures were performed, resulting in 37,136 deaths at a cost of $122 billion (using 1974 dollars).

While it is difficult to obtain accurate statistics when studying unnecessary surgery, Dr. Leape conceded in 1989 that perhaps 30 percent of controversial surgeries (including cesarean section, tonsillectomy, appendectomy, hysterectomy, gastrectomy for obesity, breast implants, and elective breast implants) are unnecessary. In 1974, the Congressional Committee on Interstate and Foreign Commerce held hearings on unnecessary surgery. It found that 17.6 percent of recommendations for surgery were not confirmed by a second opinion. The House Subcommittee on Oversight and Investigations extrapolated these figures and estimated that, on a nationwide basis, there were 2.4 million unnecessary surgeries performed annually, resulting in 11,900 deaths at an annual cost of $3.9 billion.

According to the Healthcare Cost and Utilization Project within the Agency for Healthcare Research and Quality(13), in 2001 the 50 most common medical and surgical procedures were performed approximately 41.8 million times in the U.S.

Using the 1974 House Subcommittee on Oversight and Investigations' figure of 17.6 percent as the percentage of unnecessary surgical procedures, and extrapolating from the death rate in 1974, produces nearly 7.5 million (7,489,718) unnecessary procedures and a death rate of 37,136, at a cost of $122 billion (using 1974 dollars).

The Health Services Research Journal reports that in 1995, researchers conducted a similar analysis of back surgery procedures, using the 1974 "unnecessary surgery percentage" of 17.6. Testifying before the Department of Veterans Affairs, they estimated that of the 250,000 back surgeries performed annually in the US at a hospital cost of $11,000 per patient, the total number of unnecessary back surgeries approaches 44,000, costing as much as $484 million.(75

Like prescription drug use driven by television advertising, unnecessary surgeries are escalating. Media-driven surgery such as gastric bypass for obesity and all but endorsed by Hollywood celebrities, seduces obese people into thinking this procedure is safe and sexy.

Unnecessary surgeries have even been marketed online. A study in Spain declared that 20-25 percent of total surgical practice represents unnecessary operations.

According to data from the National Center for Health Statistics for 1979 to 1984, the total number of surgical procedures increased 9% while the number of surgeons grew 20%. The study notes that the large increase in the number of surgeons was not accompanied by a parallel increase in the number of surgeries performed. The researchers wondered aloud how an excess of surgeons would handle the comparatively smaller surgical caseload.

From 1983 to 1994, however, the incidence of the 10 most commonly performed surgical procedures jumped 38 percent to 7,929,000 from 5,731,000 cases. By 1994, cataract surgery was the most common procedure with more than 2 million operations, followed by cesarean section (858,000 procedures) and inguinal hernia operations (689,000 procedures).

Knee arthroscopy procedures increased a staggering 153 percent while prostate surgery declined 29 percent. The list of iatrogenic complications from surgery is as long as the list of procedures themselves. One study examined catheters that were inserted to deliver anesthetic into the epidural space around the spinal nerves for lower cesarean section, abdominal surgery, or prostate surgery. JAMA Surgery reported that, in some cases, non-sterile techniques during catheter insertion resulted in serious infections, even leading to limb paralysis.

In one review of the literature, the authors noted "a significant rate of overutilization of coronary angiography, coronary artery surgery, cardiac pacemaker insertion, upper gastrointestinal endoscopies, carotid endarterectomies, back surgery, and pain-relieving procedures."

A 1987 JAMA study found the following significant levels of inappropriate surgery:

• 17 percent of coronary angiography procedures
• 32 percent of carotid endarterectomy procedures
• 17 percent of upper gastrointestinal tract endoscopy procedures.(82)

Based on the HCUP statistics provided by the government for 2001, 697,675 upper gastrointestinal endoscopies (usually entailing biopsy) were performed

- 142,401 endarterectomies
- 719,949 coronary angiographies

Extrapolating the JAMA study's inappropriate surgery rates to 2001 produces:

- 118,604 unnecessary endoscopy procedures
- 45,568 unnecessary endarterectomies, and
- 122,391 unnecessary coronary angiographies (are all forms of medical iatrogenesis)

So, here is the problem. If you have made it this far in this book, you will find it just goes on and on. Sadly the American population still is not totally awake.

The good news is there are folks like you and me who are awake. When I was in graduate school at Florida State University I attended more than a few classes with future medical doctors. Without exception they were all great at memorization. There were a few with common sense. But the vast majority could not think outside of the box. In other words, they always followed the same template. That's okay, as long as the template is correct.

But, here is the problem: the medical template is broken in our country. The medical system is broken. Its primary function has become to treat symptoms not the underlying problem. Let me give you an example. If you have a headache you do not have a deficiency of aspirin. The aspirin only treats the symptom. There may be a serious underlying cause like a brain tumor. That's what traditional medicine has been trained to do, treat symptoms.

Very rarely does a medical doctor try and figure out "What is the underlying cause of this condition". That is simply because many of the students who are accepted into medical school are good at memorizing and taking standardized tests. But sadly they have difficulty in developing concrete rational thought and problem solving as part of their practice. If they do wake up and start asking questions and jump out of the box, they run the risk of losing their license.

The good news is more and more folks like you are waking up. When I first started my practice thirty-three years ago, I thought everyone was asleep. But, thanks to the internet and some TV shows who are not afraid to tell the truth, more and more of us are waking up. All I can say is, it is about time.

Victory Over
7 PMS and Menopause
by Sharon Broer

Wouldn't it be wonderful to be able to go through your 20's, 30's, 40's and 50's never experiencing menstrual cramps, mood swings, blotting, weight gain and hot flashes? That would only be possible if we lived in a perfect world, and obviously we don't. But, I do have some good news ladies. There are healthy and natural solutions to these hormonal challenges that we face throughout our lives.

God has created our bodies in such an amazing and complex way and most of our body functions rely on one word: HORMONES. You might say, hormones "call the shots." They come in all shapes and sizes, helping the body to grow, mature and maintain itself. Next time you feel you can't live with these special messengers, remember, "You can't live without them."

My husband, Ted, and I have been blessed with a wonderful family; one pre-teen daughter, one teen daughter, one teen son, one 25 year old son, and one 25 year old, beautiful daughter-in-law. Add one menopausal mother (I'm now 56), and I guess you could say we are experiencing hormones from A to Z.

Hormones are our bodies' chemical messengers. The endocrine glands, which include the pituitary, the adrenals, the pancreas, the pineal, the thymus and the thyroid, all produce hormones. It is astonishing to me how important hormones are to our overall well-being and our health.

The hormone estrogen is mainly produced in the ovaries, but some estrogens are produced in smaller amounts by the adrenal, the breast and the liver glands. Fat cells also produce estrogen.

Years before we start our first menstrual cycle through the years ending menopause, our bodies are continually experiencing hormonal changes. These changes are directly affected by four nutritional and lifestyle variables: diet and nutrient deficiencies, exercise, sleep and stress.

HORMONES
AND LIFESTYLE

Diet plays such a big role in overcoming PMS and menopause symptoms. Cutting back on salty and caffeine products will help with blotting and irritability. Reducing processed foods and sugar contributes to reducing mood swings. Eating more whole fresh foods like veggies, brown rice, lean chicken and fish and some beef also play a big role in overcoming PMS symptoms. My motto is to eat CLEAN, GREEN, LEAN and good PROTEIN. We bring our whey protein in from New Zealand (because it is so pure), that is in our Fit Food Protein. I love it and it reminds me of the Carnation Instant Breakfast I grew up on. We make milk shakes with frozen (peeled) ripe bananas, organic milk and chocolate Fit Food, which even my children love. This is also a healthy alternative when those chocolate cravings go wild. Remember, if it's not in the house, you can't eat it. It is also very important to eat more organic dairy like Greek yogurt and non-homogenized milk. If you buy plain yogurt and sweeten it with Stevia, you cut out so many more calories. For a chocolate pudding replacement, mix some chocolate Fit Food in with your yogurt. It is heavenly! Visit us on Facebook or YouTube to watch our cooking and workout videos.

Exercise is important for weight maintenance (or loss), improved muscle mass, increased bone density, and an overall feeling of well-being. Even just getting moderate exercise a few times a week will increase circulation and improve your overall outlook.

Sleep, or I should say enough sleep, is critical especially during your monthly cycle. Make it a priority over late night plans. I'm sure your friends will understand and appreciate it. Try to get in bed thirty minutes earlier than usual and naps, even "cat naps" always help with those irritability issues. Remember, your body is more fatigued this time of the month.

Stress serves a useful purpose when it is for a short duration. The hormones release a flight or fight God-given response that can save your life, or the life of another, like snatching up a child to prevent them from being hit by an oncoming bike or car, or running as fast as you can when you find yourself in a pasture full of cows and realize one of them is a bull.

When a stress response is constantly or frequently activated in your body, like dealing with an irritating boss or a disobedient child, your menstrual and menopause symptoms will become more noticeable. For example, your menstrual period may become heavier and your hot flashes may increase in frequency and duration. If your body is remaining in a constant stress mode, the hormone cortisol is released and is stored as belly fat. I hate to admit it, but knowing this has helped we work harder on controlling my temper. Hey, at least I'm honest.

Something as simple as laughing can be the best prescription for reducing stress. God already knew that when He tells us in Proverbs 17:22, "A cheerful heart is like good medicine." Research has proven, when you laugh your muscles relax, your stress hormones decrease, your immune function improves, your blood pressure lowers and your blood sugar levels lower. Speaking about laughter, have you ever wondered why the word menstrual and menopause start with "men" even though it's "women's stuff? " Figure that one out.

PMS PREMEMSTRUAL SYNDROME

While not every woman experiences PMS, about 75% to 85% report having at least one of the following symptoms: cramping, bloating, or irritability each month. Being the mother of two girls, who God has made completely different, I have observed that temperament (or personality) plays a major role in how these symptoms are handled. One personality may be so fun- loving and optimistic that if she experiences any PMS symptoms, I would seldom know it. On the other hand, the other personality may not be as optimistic which would in turn cause more complaining and irritability. I tell my girls that we do everything in the natural for these symptoms, but complaining just makes things worse. Then I quote Proverbs 18:21: "...that life and death are in the power of the tongue." Attitude is everything!

There are 5 ways to know if you have PMS...

1. Everyone around you has an attitude problem.
2. You find yourself adding chocolate to all your food.
3. The clothes dryer has shrunk every pair of jeans you own.
4. Your husband (or boyfriend) is agreeing with everything you are saying.
5. You are using your cell phone to dial up every bumper sticker that reads, "How's my driving, dial 1-800-...-..."

I remember when I had my monthly cycle and some months my husband would ask me, "Am I getting Sharon A or Sharon B today?" Then we would laugh, but I think he was serious. That is about the same time we started working on our Natural PMS Support program. I tweaked it over the years until I got the results I needed. Now even my daughter-in-law is enjoying the benefits of this program with great results.

PMS Support Program

1. **PMS Support** — this is a comprehensive blend of Native and American herbs traditionally used to provide balance and support for a healthy menstrual cycle. By convention, menstrual cycles are counted from the first day of menstrual bleeding. Most women take 1 -3 capsules mid-cycle, approximately day 14 through day 2 of their period. If symptoms are more frequent women may take during entire cycle. Except for cramping, it may take more than one cycle to experience results. Can be taken with or without food.

2. **Ossomag** — this is an excellent calcium, magnesium and D3 formula. Sugar robs calcium out of the teeth and bones. Calcium and magnesium helps your body to relax, especially your muscles. Calcium taken at night helps you sleep better.

3. **Iron Glycinate** — loss of blood each month means loss of iron. Low iron levels can lead to fatigue, anemia and low blood pressure. Most iron supplements are almost impossible for the body to absorb. That's why Healthmasters offers Iron Glycinate. This patented form of iron uses the amino acid glycine which is one of the two starting materials the body uses to synthesize hemoglobin. Therefore, Iron Glycinate contributes two key factors. This form of iron has higher bioavailability, lower toxicity, less food reactivity, less food interactions and has a longer shelf life than any other common form of iron. I have had so many women call our office so excited about the results they have gotten from using this natural iron source. They also are happy to no longer feel the nausea they were experiencing from the iron supplements they were taking.

4. **Healthmasters B Complex** — this helps tremendously with irritability and mood swings by regulating the nervous system. It also helps support stress related function. I call this my "energy vitamin."

5. **5-HTP (5 hydrozytrytopan)** — this is a drug-free amino acid derived from a plant that naturally increases the bodies level of serotonin, the chemical messenger that affects emotions, behavior, appetite and sleep. This also helps promote a more positive outlook and greater appetite control. I call this my "happy vitamin."

6. **Sublingual Melatonin** — this helps to maintain healthy sleep patterns as well as antioxidant and immune activities. Helps with sleep when restless and cramping.

MENOPAUSE

This is one of those inquisitive subjects I would like to ask God about when I get to heaven. I'm sure women (and men) that are in their mid -forties and early fifties feel the same way. Menopause means "the end of monthly cycles," starting in the early to mid-forties and ending in the mid to late fifties. Ladies, this part of our life is a "Catch 22." We are excited to no longer have to deal with monthly cycles and think of the money we will be saving no longer buying feminine hygiene products, (unless teenage girls are still at home). Life is "going good", then, from out of nowhere these foreign internal feelings that are like standing in front of a fireplace with a roaring fire on a hot August afternoon in Florida, creep up on us. I once heard a joke that said, "Don't think of it as hot flashes; think of it as your inner child playing with matches."

It's funny, but every "hormone hostage" (husband, boyfriend), knows that there are days in the month when all a man has to do is open his mouth and he takes his life into his own hands. We have found, as a family, when we can joke about this "menopause stuff", every now and then, our home becomes more peaceful. Life is easier when we can laugh at ourselves from time to time, and lighten up and not take life so seriously.

Now at the age 56, I have the stories to tell, the experiences to share, and best of all, the products to help you enter this part of your life with excitement, enjoyment, vitality, energy and breakthrough health.

In my early forties, my husband, Ted retired from the "Success" speaking circuit. After being on the road and flying around the country week after week for years, we decided to finish our family. Our first child was ten and my time was running out. We now have four wonderful miracles from God, and each one is incredibility different.

During this time of my life I found myself in a very unusual situation. I was raising one teen and three "little ones" and at the same time experiencing symptoms of this new part of life called menopause. My hormones became the "seven dwarves of menopause": itchy, snappy, sweaty, sleepy, bloated, forgetful and psychotic.

Like so many other women my age, I decided to have my hormone levels checked. I was informed that my testosterone level was extremely low. This explained my low blood pressure and fatigue. Being a very active mother of four, homeschooling, working out 5 days a week and being a partner with my husband running our business, Healthmasters, I had to do something. I decided to go the route of natural hormone therapy through a compounding pharmacy. I was so excited that I would have more energy, and I did. But one problem, my testosterone levels were not monitored properly, and I ended up with levels 100 times higher than normal. It was incredible how strong I became with much more definition in my muscles. I was burning body fat with legs that looked like they did in my twenties. But, looks are not everything. I became very empowered, intense, less patient, and yes, very type A. Being married to a type A German, how do you think that worked out? If my husband said, "The car is red," I would say, "no, it's not, it's blue-red." I became very argumentative and lost all my reasoning skills.

There were days when Ted would ask me to please go to my mother's house just to give my family a break. Once we discovered my testosterone levels were at an insane level I knew we had to develop a natural menopause protocol to help women avoid what I had gone through. We have tweaked this program, with me being the test subject, and now have a natural menopause protocol that we have used to help women around the world. It's so nice to be balanced with very few hot flashes, even living in Florida. I no longer experience that "down" or depressed feeling as long as I follow the program daily. My energy levels are amazing with perfect blood pressure. I weigh two pounds more than I did when I married my husband. I work out 5 – 6 days a week, doing stretching, cardio and weight resistance training. I share my workouts and other informative videos on Facebook and YouTube.

Menopause Support Program

1. **Menopause Support** – this formula, using selected herbs and nutrients support the adrenal glands, relaxation and overall well-being. Also, this may beneficially influence estrogen receptor function:
2. **5-HTP CR (5 hydroxytryophan)** – this is a drug-free amino acid derived form a plant that naturally increases the bodies level of serotonin, the chemical messenger that affects emotions, behavior, appetite and sleep. This helps promote a more positive outlook and greater appetite control. As I said earlier, I call this my "happy vitamin."
3. **Healthmasters B-Complex** – this is important for the support of the adrenal hormone production and stress related function. As mentioned earlier, I call this my "stress and energy vitamin."
4. **Healthmasters Cod Liver Oil** – this is liquid and though it's not the best tasting supplement I take, I won't go a day without it. This is great for brain function, inflammation, and it helps regulate mood swings. It also helps overcome that "depressed", down feeling. I take 2 tablespoons every day.
5. **DHEA Cream** – this is the mother of all hormones. It helps to regulate all other hormones (including testosterone), which is the hormone that burns body fat. It supports healthy cholesterol and glucose levels, and

helps support healthy sexual function. It provides your body with the material to maintain healthy levels of serotonin. Low levels of serotonin may result in depression, obesity and carb cravings. I use one pump a day alternating inner thighs and inner arms. Before using the creams, I recommend getting a saliva or blood test and follow the advice of your doctor.

6. **Healthmasters Progesterone Cream** — this has been formulated with the finest natural bio identical progesterone with polytoestrogens and with no parabens. For women entering menopause, decreasing supplies of progesterone may cause intense hot flashes, mood swings, weight gain, excessive vaginal dryness, greatly diminished or loss of libido and an overall decline in health and vitality. I use one pump a day alternating inner thighs and inner arms. Before using cream I recommend getting a saliva or blood test and follow the advice of your doctor.

7. **Sublingual Melatonin** — this helps maintain healthy sleep patterns as well as antioxidant and immune activities.

Today, we are living in a world of nutrient depleted foods. Even when we try to eat clean and healthy, it is impossible for our body to get everything it needs to function at top optimum health. Supplementation has become a necessity. I am so thankful, thirty years ago when my husband and I birthed *Healthmasters* that we have been blessed to help so many people from all walks of life, all over the world. I am even more thankful that through the experiences we personally have gone through, we can honestly tell you, first hand, that our programs get results.

8 | The Dangers of Immunizations

98 Million Polio Vaccinations
May Have Contained Cancer Virus:

I have warned you for years about the dangers of immunizations. This confirms why I think and believe you should never immunize yourself nor any members of your family.

98 million Americans may have received one or more doses of polio vaccine within an 8-year span when a proportion of the vaccine was contaminated with a cancer causing polyomavirus called SV40. It has been estimated that 10-30 million Americans could have received an SV40 contaminated dose of the vaccine. Like other polyomaviruses, SV40 is a DNA virus that has been found to cause tumors and cancer. Really? So they are openly coming out now and saying these vaccines contained cancer cells.

Now please understand in 1955 there was roughly a population of only 166 million people. Meaning that roughly 20% of the entire USA could have been given this cancer virus! And, with the current processed foods loaded with chemical ingredients and GMO's, this very well could play a pivotal role in why so many people seem to get cancer in their 50's. This is why we recommend that everyone takes the Ultimate Multiple Vitamin to replace all the vitamins and minerals we no longer get in our food.

The SV40 is believed to suppress the transcriptional properties of the tumor-suppressing genes in humans through the SV40 Large T-antigen and SV40 Small T-antigen. Mutated genes may contribute to uncontrolled cellular proliferation, leading to cancer.

Michele Carbone, Assistant Professor of Pathology at Loyola University in Chicago, has recently isolated fragments of the SV-40 virus in human bone cancers called osteosarcoma and in a lethal form of lung cancer called mesothelioma.

Dr. Michele Carbone even openly acknowledged that HIV/AIDS was spread by the hepatitis B vaccine produced by Merck & Co. during the early 1970's. This was the very first time since the initial transmissions took place in 1972-74, that a top leading expert in this field of vaccine manufacturing and testing has openly admitted the Merck & Co. liability for AIDS.

This startling disclosure was brought up during discussions of polio vaccines contaminated with the SV40 virus, which caused cancer in nearly **every** species vaccinated by the contaminated injection. Many authorities are now admitting some of the world's cancers came from the Salk and Sabin polio vaccines, and hepatitis B vaccines, produced in monkeys and chimps.

It has been said that the lung cancer known as mesothelioma is a result of asbestos exposure, but research reveals that 50% of the current mesothelioma lung cancer being treated no longer occurs due to asbestos but rather the SV-40 virus contained in the polio vaccination

Now, are you ready for this? The SV-40 virus has now been detected in tumors removed from people never given the contaminated vaccine, leading some researchers to conclude that those infected by the vaccine might actually be spreading SV40. This means it is possible that the virus could be transferred from person to person or from parent to children.

To make things even worse, it was found later that the technique used to inactivate the polio virus in the injectable vaccine, was through means of **formaldehyde**, which did not reliably kill SV40. Formaldehyde? Really? Yes, the exact substance they put into cadavers at the morgue. This just continues to show you why you should think twice before getting vaccinated.

To keep your immune system healthy and ready for any attack, stay loaded up on Healthmasters

- Excellent C,
- Immune support DF,
- Ultimate D3-5000,
- Viragraphics,
- or simply order our Flu prevention kit.

The products listed above can be very helpful along with our Healthmasters Ultimate Immune Booster which contains a patented Broccoli seed extract that helps to strengthen the immune system.

9 Simple Trick to Turn Back Your Aging Clock

I'm 57 years young and I feel great. I have, however, noticed something; I am no longer a teenager. When I eat something I shouldn't (NEWS FLASH-I do that occasionally), or I don't get enough sleep, I can feel it.

From the minute we are born we begin to grow and develop. This process continues until our mid- twenties. Then something amazing happens. Our bodies begin to age. Sadly, for so many people, their best days are probably behind them, if they are over 25. But, most of us really don't care about the aging process until we can see it in the mirror or until it begins to affect us personally. Suddenly we look in the mirror and we have new wrinkles, feel new aches and pains, have body fat gain, muscle loss, fatigue, high blood pressure, feel always tired, and our memory starts failing. This list can go on and on.

Well, growing older, we soon realize, is part of the life process. But, I have realized that sitting around feeling horrible and waiting to die doesn't have to be part of life. Break through science is showing us, through applied research, that we are all very much in control of our aging process if, and only if, you decide to take action and do something about aging. If you take action, I believe that you too can become one of those "Blessed" people who have tremendous energy, vitality, and top mental activity well into your 50's, 60's, 70's, 80's, and 90's and beyond. Remember, in the old testament Moses lived to be 120 and was as sharp as a tack.

Has the fountain of youth really been discovered? Several years ago it was shown that systematic under- eating helped to extend the life span. The problem is it's a very depriving life style. You are always hungry.

Years ago I told you that we had developed **HGH Stimulate** to help the pituitary gland release HGH and really slow down the aging process? Well guess what? We have now developed another product that activates the anti- aging genes, fights free radicals, promotes body fat loss, protects the cardiovascular system, helps to balance blood, fights infections, helps support the immune system, protects the brain, and as for me personally, greatly improved my mental acuity. Remember I take a lot of supplements. Most of the other ones I have tried or done clinical research on do not work. That's why you never hear of them.

This new product is called Reservatrol Plus.

WOW! This product is amazing!!!!! Exciting new research has shown that Reservatrol actually mimics the effect of a low calorie diet. These effects include increasing in lifespan up to 70%. Overwhelming research from leading institutions around the world points to the same conclusion, Reservatrol has the potential to extend human life.

It actually works by activating the very genes that control the aging process. It actually switches on the genes effectively slowing aging and protecting against the degenerative diseases of aging.

By the way, the research is so overwhelmingly convincing that the drug companies have taken note. One has actually spent 720 million trying to develop a patented form so they can control it.

The problem with Reservatrol is that everyone has jumped on the bandwagon and they are producing cheap, chemical laden, bad ingredient products that don't work. Most companies use the inferior CIS form, not the potent trans form of Reservatrol Plus. Also the product must be standardized, otherwise you really don't know the potency. **All of Health Masters supplements are nutraceuticals' grade**. The Health Masters label is the best you can buy, PERIOD! Plus, we even add 250 mg of Quercetin, the strongest antioxidant known. To obtain the purest Reservatrol possible we use only the purest most potent natural extracts possible. I take these every day.

So here's my Top Mental Activity, Top Energy, Slow- Down- The Aging Process- Arsenal:

Reservatrol Plus	Massively slows down aging, inhibits Breast and Prostate Cancer, helps to obtain top mental activity. THIS IS AN AMAZING PRODUCT!
HGH Stimulate	Burns body fat, increases human growth hormone, lowers Blood Pressure, increases strength and Libido.
Ultimate Multiple	Best Multiple Vitamin on the planet. PERIOD!
Cortico B5 B6	Bathes the Brain in B5 B6. YOU CAN FEEL THIS ONE.
B Complex	Helps the body produce energy.
Excellent C	Helps maintain healthy collagen, the cellular glue which helps to maintain skin elasticity.
Cod Liver Oil	Thins the blood and provides Omega 3 fats...THIS IS A CRITICAL PRODUCT
Super Potent E	Helps blood flow to Brain and keeps your Heart strong!
Ultimate D3-5000	Does just about everything, plus it's a real Immune System booster.
Fit Food Protein	Provides the essential amino acids your body needs, plus it tastes great.

All of these high quality supplements can also be purchased by calling my office at 1-800-726-1834.

10 | Bisphenol-A BPA

I have written about this several times: The intentional use of BPA in plastic food wrap and containers.

This is something the United States Government should have never allowed.

Not only have they allowed it, they refuse to remove this feminizing cancer- causing poison

from our food supply. We have an estrogen blocker called **Healthmasters Ultimate Estrogen Blocker**.

I highly recommend that everyone who has any potential exposure to these environmental poisons start taking this product as soon as possible..

For those of you who like to read the "proof through research," you are going to love this!

If you have any questions please call my office. And yes, we still answer the phone 800- 726- 1834.

The Environmental Protection Agency (EPA) has a list of over 400 known chemicals that cause neurotoxic effect on the brain. The effect is in the brain's ability to grow and develop properly. Bisphenol-A is one of the chemicals on this list!

Please go online and type in the links I have provided here, if you desire further information:

EPA Building a Database of Developmental Neurotoxicants:
http://www.epa.gov/ncct/toxcast/files/summit/48P%20Mundy%20TDAS.pdf

After becoming aware of the disclosures made by the EPA let's go over to the Johns Hopkins Bloomberg School of Public Health where we will learn how BPA affects our bodies and the brains of laboratory animals:

http://www.jhsph.edu/publichealthnews/articles/2008/goldman_schwab_bpa.html

With 6 billion pounds of BPA being produced each year it is no wonder why it is in 93% of people tested. Money is definitely a factor in the decisions of governments to ban or limit the import/export of Bisphenol-A. For instance, here you can see the United States government telling France that they cannot ban BPA because it will hurt U.S exports:

http://experimentalvaccines.org/Sweden

Scientific America reported on April 1, 2012, that the U.S. will opt Not to Ban BPA in canned foods:

http://www.scientificamerican.com/article.cfm?id=us-opts-not-to-ban-bpa-in-can

Science Daily reported that: Bisphenol -A Exposure In Pregnant Mice Permanently Changes DNA Of Offspring:

http://www.sciencedaily.com/releases/2009/06/090610124428.htm

Notes:
- Always buy bottled water in glass.
- Never store water in plastic.
- Use a **Healthmasters distiller**!
- More on water in the aluminum chapter

Senile Dementia and Alzheimer's: Know the Truth

11

If someone asked you to name an environmental hazard that personally affects you, chances are you wouldn't know what to say, right? Wrong! Next time you think of environmental hazards, consider this: A few years back, I heard of a farmer whose central nervous system had been severely damaged as a result of having been splashed with a pesticide. After the incident, even though he showered in order to rid his skin of the contaminant, he became ill. His doctor gave a drug that typically reverses the chemical process of the pesticide but instead, his condition worsened: the nerves in his arms and legs continued to deteriorate, and he suffered from stuttering, loss of coordination and had difficulty organizing his thoughts. His doctor was baffled, so he started reading up on the neurological damage in humans caused by that particular pesticide and pesticides, in general. As a result of his research on the subject of neurotoxicology, he ultimately came to the conclusion that remains true today: We live in a sea of toxins.

The Connection between Aluminum and Dementia

Toxic metals in our environment produce a slow degeneration of our nervous system. One metal, aluminum, is the third most common element on earth and has been known to be toxic to the brain since 1911. Right now, if I were you I would be wondering why I hadn't been told this information. In reality, until the last few decades, it has been pretty much ignored. Until recently, scientists didn't think aluminum was a significant problem because they knew it was poorly absorbed in the GI tract. The reason aluminum even became an issue was that large amounts were being added to antacids. This, in my opinion, as you read on, is one of the primary causes of neurodegenerative diseases like Alzheimer's. I will be talking of more on this later. Research shows that certain food components, such as citrate and malate (organic acids), can increase the absorption of aluminum as much as six times the normal rate. This means that all citrus fruits, such as lemons, grapefruit, and oranges, dramatically increase the absorption of aluminum from the GI tract and increase its entry into the brain. Which is why adding lemon in their black tea is a bad idea: black tea has very high levels of aluminum and the citrate from the lemon significantly increases its absorption in the GI tract. People with Alzheimer's disease and Down syndrome also have a much higher level of aluminum absorption. Studies show that injecting small doses of aluminum salts into the brain of animals can cause the neurons to degenerate and lead to some of the changes seen with Alzheimer's disease. It has been shown that adding aluminum to drinking water led to accumulations of the aluminum in the very same areas of the brain affected in Alzheimer's disease. Ultimately, someone realized that aluminum was being added to drinking water systems in the U.S. Once the incidence of Alzheimer's dementia in areas with aluminum in public drinking water was compared to areas with aluminum-free water systems, people could see a significantly higher incidence of dementia in areas with public water systems with added aluminum. Later it was discovered that aluminum toxicity occurred in concentrations that were quite small, and that aluminum was accumulating in restricted areas of the brain, rather than the entire organ. Further studies using highly sensitive testing in these specific areas confirmed that people with Alzheimer's have had significantly higher brain aluminum levels. Now it seems that we are also getting aluminum from above. Apparently the government has in its infinite wisdom — or should I say stupidity — decided to combat global warming by using aluminum oxide and barium oxide as a reflective agent in the upper atmosphere, or so the story goes . . . I can't seem to get a straight answer from public officials as to what they're actually spraying in the atmosphere. There are some official government statements online, but they're few and far between. All I know is this: aluminum is really bad for your brain and barium is really bad for your immune system. So I hope and pray that these are not the compounds being used. The biggest concern I have with this is that we have had multiple hair analysis come into my office with extremely high levels of barium and aluminum. These hair analysis are so extreme that Sharon and I have also sent in samples of our hair to see if our aluminum and barium levels are high. I suggest that all of you do this. (Health Masters' Hair Analysis) Also, we have increased our intake of our oral chelation product (Health Masters' Chelation Therapy) which binds and helps to remove metals. Please call my office for details on how to have a hair analysis done and to get more information on oral chelation. Also, remember to use or get a water distiller (Health Masters' Water Distiller 8800), which takes the aluminum and barium out of the water. Call 1-800-726-1834 with any questions. I'd have a hard time believing any of this if I had not seen the jets here in central Florida leaving a white trail of spray on almost a daily basis. These, by the way, are not contrails. Contrails dissipate a few thousand yards behind a jet. The spray which looks like smoke takes hours to dissipate. In fact, back in 1998, Florida had a major outbreak of Mediterranean fruit flies. The state was concerned for the citrus industry so they decided to combat the infestation with Malathion. Now here's where things get crazy: They didn't spray just the orange groves. They sprayed a known neurotoxin on everything and everyone in central Florida. I still remember standing outside my home looking up helplessly as a DC3 flew overhead releasing a cloud of this poison. It wasn't until a consumer group sued the State of Florida did it finally stop by decree of a court order. After that incident, there's nothing much that the government does that surprises me.

Aluminum — Straight from the Faucet

Until an incident in the 1980s, the connection between dementia and aluminum still wasn't taken seriously. Then, doctors in several hospitals noticed that some of their dialysis patients developed unusual symptoms, including muscle spasms, hallucinations, and a rapid onset of dementia. But before answers could be found, many of those patients died. It was later discovered that all of the affected patients had high levels of aluminum in their blood and brains, and the source of that aluminum? The tap water used for their dialysis. It was common practice for treatment plants to add aluminum to tap water to remove particulate matter. Especially, as aluminum is removed from the body primarily by the kidneys. Unfortunately, since dialysis patients have no kidney function, the aluminum in their body was rising to toxic levels. Since that incident, other cases of long-term ingestion of aluminum-containing antacids in patients with poor kidney function have appeared, including the use of an aluminum composite plate in a brain operation. And in each case, before dying, each patient developed seizures, confusion, and dementia. Examination of their brains didn't show the typical pathological findings of Alzheimer's disease, only widespread degeneration of selected areas of the brain. It is important to remember that these were acute exposures — exposure to high levels of aluminum in a short period of time. Using animal test subjects in studies which mimicked normal, daily exposure to lower doses of aluminum did show changes similar to Alzheimer's disease and Lou Gehrig's disease (ALS), another neurodegenerative condition. The conclusion: even trace amounts of aluminum, like that found in a glass of water, readily entered the brains of animals.

The Effect of Aluminum on the Brain

Aluminum damages the brain in many ways:

1. By dramatically increasing the accumulation of free radicals and lipid peroxidation products in the brain.

2. By displacing iron from its normal carrier proteins, transferrin and ferritin, and causing free iron to accumulate in the blood and brain, leading to high levels of free radicals and lipid peroxidation products (oxidative stress).

3. By interfering with adenosine triphosphate-dependent enzymes (ATP-dependent) that carry out the critical function of energy transfer between brain cells.

4. By interfering with a number of important enzymes and cell processes that are crucial to brain function. Okay. So now you've heard all the scientific jargon.

Here's what it all means: Aluminum is a brain and central nervous system poison. It basically makes you stupid and incapable of continuing to function as a responsible adult. I know that sounds harsh . . . and it should . . . because it's the truth. This is one of the reasons I've pleaded with my readers for 25 years to purchase one of the distillers (Health Masters' Water Distiller 8800) on my website so they can remove the aluminum from their drinking water. It doesn't matter if you have well or good city water — I guarantee all of it has compounds and other stuff that you should not put into your body. Because aluminum is so prevalent in the ecosystem, it has to be manually removed from drinking water via distillation. I used to drink ice tea in restaurants, no longer. Why? Simply because they don't use distilled water to make the tea and you really have no way of knowing what's in the water, period. What I do now is order bottled water, add fresh lemon and sweeten it with Stevia (Health Masters' Stevia). Sometimes I even bring my own distilled water in a Voss bottle. If the restaurant complains, I tell them to add the cost of bottled water to my bill. I understand that they have to cover overhead so I don't have a problem paying for my own water. The next reality is that I NEVER buy distilled water in a plastic container. The plastic compounds will actually leech into the water. I prefer storing water in glass. When my family travels in our motor home, we bring one gallon glass containers (like an apple juice jug) full of distilled water along. When we run out we refill them by going to a grocery store and using a Reverse Osmosis machine. It's not as good as distillation, but its close enough. If you are forced to buy bottled water, always buy the hardest plastic available, and do not buy distilled in the store, period. Get a sturdy — not soft — plastic container. Trust me; the poisons released from soft plastics are horrible for you.

Aluminum and the Nervous System

One review of aluminum toxicity toward the nervous system indicates that a main toxic effect is immuno excitotoxicity. This involves triggering brain inflammation in combination with excitotoxicity. It's pretty well established that aluminum specifically targets the brain and causes it to become inflamed, which is why Alzheimer's disease, Parkinson's disease, and ALS are all considered to be inflammatory diseases and excitotoxic diseases. One of the commonly found reactions to aluminum in the brain is the activation of the brain's immune cell — the microglia. This has been found in all cases of dialysis dementia and other reported cases of aluminum toxicity. Researchers at the University of Georgia found that mice given aluminum- containing drinking water secreted higher levels of the inflammatory cytokine TNF-alpha than did those drinking aluminum-free water. TNF-alpha is primarily secreted by the microglia. This means when you drink your aluminum containing tap water, your brain secretes higher levels of inflammatory chemicals putting you at a greater risk of Alzheimer's disease. It also puts your children at risk of abnormal brain development, learning and behavioral problems. Aluminum also interferes with mitochondrial energy production and brain cells are extremely dependent on a constant supply of energy. Anything that reduces the brain's supply of energy greatly magnifies its sensitivity to excitotoxicity. Another way aluminum enhances excitotoxicity is by combining with glutamate, the excitotoxic amino acid. Unfortunately, glutamate is found in a great many foods, either as an additive or naturally occurring. The aluminum binds with the glutamate, forming an aluminum-L-glutamate complex that is highly absorbed by both the GI tract and the brain. Interestingly, a new study found that magnesium aspartate decreased the aluminum concentration in the brain cortex of rats. In another study, researchers fed rats either aluminum glutamate complex, aluminum chloride, or glutamate alone and found that the aluminum glutamate complex significantly increased brain aluminum levels over just feeding aluminum chloride alone, thus reaching high levels in the key areas of the brain:

- The hippocampus
- The Occipito-parietal cortex
- The Cerebellum10. The aluminum-glutamate complex appeared to make the blood-brain barrier more permeable to aluminum. From these studies it appears that aluminum, either as a salt or combined with glutamate or citrate, triggers brain inflammation and excitotoxicity, which over decades leads to a slow degeneration of specific areas of the brain and spinal cord.

The Aluminum/Vaccine Connection

Amid heated debates over the cause of autism, much attention focused on the mercury additive, thimerosal. Yet, somehow the medical establishment ignored 100 years of studies clearly demonstrating the toxicity of mercury, a known neurotoxin. Then, sympathetic scientists flooded the medical literature with "studies" that found no harm at all from mercury/thimerosal, but stated that it may actually improve one's IQ. (This by the way is INSANE). Of course, everyone who knew better preferred to hide in the shadows rather than point out the glaring flaws in these 'studies'. Vaccination had now become the subject of political correctness, still hiding in the shadows of arguing over vaccinations — the obvious toxicity of aluminum. Research had previously demonstrated that aluminum was an accumulative neurotoxin, even in small concentrations. It had also been demonstrated that aluminum had a tendency to concentrate in the hippo-campus, an area of the brain vital to critical functions including:

- Learning
- Memory
- Emotions.

The other two areas of the nervous system that were known to be extremely sensitive to aluminum toxicity and to concentrate aluminum are the mid brain and the motor neurons of the motor cortex and spinal cord.

Brain Development Implications

It's neither a surprise nor coincidence that aluminum concentrates in areas of the brain associated with early childhood neurodevelopment, and in those areas associated with three major neurodegenerative diseases — Alzheimer's, Parkinson's, and ALS. Additionally, it also concentrates in the myelin covering of neural pathways, linking it to another degenerative disease — multiple sclerosis. By the way, for nearly a century, aluminum has been added to vaccines; its purpose is to stimulate the immune system to react against the organism in the vaccine. When injected into the muscles, the aluminum forms a complex with invading organisms (like the influenza virus). This complex then attracts the body's immune cells which react to the aluminum-influenza complex by generating antibodies. At the same time, the body makes a genetic record of the invading organism for future reference. Or, at least that's how it's supposed to work. You know I when tell you something it has to really anger you. I know just writing and researching does that to me. I knew this stuff was bad but it just keeps getting worse. The sad part is — the government has this information, yet they refuse to stop the mass poisoning.

How Vaccinations Affect the Immune System:

Actually, how the immune system works is still largely a mystery. Yet, there is growing evidence that our current vaccination policy is, ironically, weakening our immune systems. What most of the public doesn't know is that recurring natural exposure to childhood viruses not only keeps our immune systems resistant to infections, it also provides resistance to cancer. In one well-researched study on the neurotoxic effects of aluminum adjuvant in vaccines, the data on the prevalence of autism spectrum disorders recorded from 1991 to 2008 was analyzed and correlated with the total aluminum dose from all vaccines mandated by the CDC for children up to age six. That was also done for the United Kingdom, Australia, Canada, Sweden, Finland, and Iceland. It's common knowledge that injected aluminum adjuvant remain at the site of the injection for years, and that aluminum is released slowly into the bloodstream and then enters other organs, including the brain. Hundreds of cases of a new disorder called macrophagic myofasciitis, which affects specialized immune cells (macrophages), have been linked to the aluminum in the muscle tissue. It has also been associated with progressive brain degeneration in children vaccinated with the tetanus and hepatitis B vaccines. The FDA has set the safe dosage limit for aluminum at 5 mcg/kg body weight per day. Below are the aluminum contents of commonly administered vaccines:

- DTaP (diphtheria, tetanus, and pertussis) — 625 mcg
- Hepatitis B — 375 mcg • Hepatitis A — 250 mcg
- Hib (haemophilus influenza type B) — 225 mcg
- PVC (pneumococcoal conjugate vaccine) — 125 mcg.

The authors of the paper found that the highest aluminum burden was given to two-month-old babies, 270 mcg/kg per day. That's almost 50 times higher than the official FDA safety limit. If we gave adults an equal dose of aluminum based on body weight, they would have to get 15 to 38 vaccines in one day. Children from the United States, the U.K., and Canada received significantly higher aluminum burdens from their vaccines than children from Scandinavian countries. This study found a strong correlation between the highest aluminum body content and the risk of developing autism. The U.K. has the most aggressive vaccine program and the highest incidence of autism in the world at 1 in every 64 births, while the rate in the U.S. is 1 in every 91 births. Unlike other countries that spread out the early vaccines, in the U.K. they're given at birth, and at 1-, 2-, 3-, and 4-months of age — an incredibly obtuse policy.

Is Aluminum Exposure Really That Widespread?

Yes, it is more widespread than you think. Consider this: From house side panels, soda cans and iPods to the deodorant you put on in the morning, thousands of products are made from aluminum; even certain medications contain an aluminum additive. And, because aluminum is added to drinking water, our plant foods are accumulating (bioaccumulating) the aluminum, so that over time the levels will continue to rise, just as we have seen with fluoride. Until recently, the main food source containing aluminum was baking powder. Biscuits, pancakes, and most baked goods have added aluminum. You can buy aluminum-free baking powder, but that version is rarely used by food processors. Salt used to contain added aluminum to prevent caking, but it has been removed from most brands. Sea salt, however, still contains aluminum. Some natural products, such as black tea, also have very high aluminum levels. The tea plant selectively extracts the aluminum from the soil and concentrates it in the leaves. (Green tea has far less aluminum, and white tea has very little.) Soy products are the number one food source for aluminum. Soybeans naturally have very high aluminum levels along with high glutamate levels. Thanks to clever marketing, Americans have been convinced to consume massive amounts of soy, including the most commonly used formula for babies. If that weren't bad enough, soy also has very high manganese levels and fluoride levels — both known neurotoxins, making soy drinks quite a neurotoxic cocktail. I have written previously, in some my mail-out newsletters , about the profound effect of the plant estrogen found in soy in feminizing baby boys and causing a variety of problems in baby girls. Do not use soy formulas. Even the American Academy of Pediatrics expressed concern about the neurotoxic level of some of the metals in soy baby formula. Studies that looked at aluminum absorption in babies exposed to aluminum found that infants absorb a considerable amount of aluminum from ingested products. So the golden rule here is simple: check labels thoroughly and if you see aluminum in the ingredients, don't buy the product.

You vs. Aluminum's Toxicity

Is there a way to battle and win against the aluminum's toxic effects? You can be sure to have a fighting chance with these four natural substances. They've been found to reduce inflammation and remove harmful metals from your body. Bee Propolis: Several studies confirm that bee propolis (a flavonoid-rich, resinous substance that bees collect from tree buds) can counteract the damaging effects of aluminum. Rats given aluminum plus propolis or propolis alone demonstrated an elevation in antioxidant enzymes and a return to normal blood lipid profiles. Propolis also has powerful anti-inflammatory properties. Ascorbic Acid-Male New Zealand rabbits in another study were given aluminum chloride and varying doses of ascorbic acid (vitamin C). Researchers found that vitamin C significantly reduced the level of free radicals generated by the aluminum and returned total lipid and cholesterol levels to normal. Chelators (Health Masters' Chelation Therapy)-A chelator is a substance used to remove excess metal from the body. The traditional pharmaceutical treatment for aluminum overload is desferrioxamine, a chelator that is administered either intramuscularly or via IV. Among its many side effects is painful swelling at the site of the injection. Feralex-G- A newer agent, appears to work best and can be taken orally. Recent studies have shown that, unlike most other aluminum chelators, Feralex-G can remove aluminum that has bound to the cell nucleus. (Aluminum tightly binds to the nucleic acid of DNA — the cause of much of its toxicity.) Combining vitamin C with Feralex-G, a process called shuttle chelation, significantly improves removal of aluminum from the cell nucleus.

How Infants React to Aluminum:

Just 4-5 mcg/kg of aluminum given to preterm infants can cause neurodevelopment problems. A study by Carolyn Gallagher and Melody Goodman (of the Stony Brook University Medical Center found that boys given the triple series of Hepatitis B vaccine from birth were significantly more likely to develop disabilities by age 9. A follow-up study of boys age 3 to 17 years old who were vaccinated in their first month had a three-fold higher risk of developing autism than did unvaccinated boys. Too bad both the media and vaccine proponents ignored this item. When challenged by this data, Dr. Paul Offit, a vocal vaccine proponent, defended the policy by saying that infant formulas often contain similar amounts of aluminum. Not quite! Studies show that only 0.25 percent of the aluminum from infant formula is absorbed in the blood, whereas 100 percent of the aluminum injected by vaccination enters the bloodstream. To date, more than one million children have been diagnosed with autism, with 24,000 new cases diagnosed each year. Interestingly, 1992 was host to the largest increase in autism diagnoses. A 189 percent jump in cases over the previous year. Why the dramatic increase that year? It turns out that six new vaccine doses were added to the vaccine schedule between 1981 and 1992, and were all given during the first two years of life — a critical period when the brain is undergoing tremendous development. The correlation between the aluminum burden from the vaccines and the incidence of autism is strong, too strong to ignore. What's more, researchers have found the same correlations in eight other countries examined. Something you'll want to consider when it's time for your children and grandchildren to be vaccinated. Current trends cannot be allowed to continue! If you're convinced that none of this actually affects you, here's the bad news: Each year adults are encouraged to submit to a number of aluminum-containing vaccines. And the effect on the adult brain can be pretty frightening:

1. First, your aging process actually reduces your brain's ability to tolerate aluminum toxicity as well as a young brain;

2. As you age, your brain becomes more inflamed, with aluminum accelerating and magnifying that inflammation;

3. Evidence indicates that aluminum worsens the effects of other toxins, such as pesticides, herbicides, mercury, cadmium, fluoride, lead, and glutamate. In essence, accumulating aluminum is making your brain age must faster.

4. Because aluminum accumulates in the parts of the brain associated with Alzheimer's, risk of early development rises substantially with exposure to aluminum.

5. All neurodegenerative diseases are associated with intense immune activation within the brain (microglia). Aluminum activates microglia, and because it accumulates within the microglia, it acts as a continuous source of activation lasting for decades.

6. Aluminum also accumulates in the motor neurons, a condition which is strongly correlated with ALS.

7. ALS used to be an extremely rare disease. That is no longer the case as the incidence of ALS has risen sharply. ALS is also characterized by intense inflammation in the nervous system. Remember the anthrax scare? Servicemen were given massive doses of the anthrax vaccine, a four dose injection, contains a total dosage of 2.4 mg of aluminum adjuvant. Since then they were found to have a two-fold higher risk of developing ALS.

8. Another link between vaccines and neurodegenerative diseases is the incredibly high incidence of multiple sclerosis following the hepatitis B vaccine in adults. The best study found a 300 percent increase in the onset of MS within two years of receiving the Hepatitis B vaccine.

Each year the drug industry releases a new set of vaccines that it promotes for good health. The industry uses the Center for Disease Control (CDC) and other federal agencies to strongly promote their widespread acceptance and use. They also use state legislation to implement mandatory vaccination for both adults and children. (Think of the vaccine requirement for college entrance). Of course, they pass a little money around to the legislators to get their laws passed. The issue of aluminum in vaccines is so very, very important and scary. If the public knew about the dangers of aluminum in vaccines, they'd be terrified. And, now most vaccines are manufactured in China, with an FDA "inspection" of these Chinese plants once every 12 years. But here's the really upsetting part — the inspectors aren't allowed to actually enter the plants! They have to accept a communist officials' word that all is 'well and safe.' If the present trend in vaccinations is allowed to continue, we'll see a nation of people so sick and mentally impaired that our survival may be compromised. It will be 9/11 on a much grander, more destructive scale!

Hungary's Toxic Horror:

Just this past fall, the Hungarian Aluminum Production and Trade Company suffered a major spill from its alumina refinery in Hungary. The spill unleashed a torrent of toxic sludge that flooded unsuspecting Hungarian towns and threatened the Danube River. The sludge, a waste product in aluminum production, contained heavy metals and is toxic if ingested. Many of the injured sustained burns as the sludge seeped through their clothes; resulting in two life-threatening conditions to the people. Company spokesmen stated that the spill contained a mixture of iron oxide, aluminum, silicon dioxide, calcium oxide, and titanium dioxide. Of those ingredients, the most toxic are iron oxide and aluminum. Iron oxide is a powerful carcinogen that promotes cancer growth, invasion, and metastasis. It is associated with degeneration of the brain and peripheral nerves, and can worsen a number of pre-existing diseases, such as pulmonary disorders, kidney disease, and heart failure. There is also evidence that iron oxide can worsen atherosclerosis — hardening of the arteries — which is a major cause of both heart attacks and strokes. As documented in this series of articles, aluminum is also a powerful toxin and can have long-term effects. Ironically, one of the effects of aluminum is release of blood iron from its protective carrier transferrin. This greatly increases the toxicity of the iron. Another worry is just how much of the aluminum was nanoparticulate aluminum — that is, aluminum that is specifically made to be of such a small size that it can easily penetrate the skin, lungs, and GI tract, entering deep into the cells. Recent studies have shown that nanoparticulate aluminum is infinitely more toxic than natural aluminum. Nanosizing products are all the rage throughout various industries — and while it can greatly improve the absorption and distribution of medications and even natural nutrients in the body, it can also increase the concentration and toxicity of toxic metals and chemicals beyond anyone's comprehension.

Forget the HPV Vaccine — Take Supplements:

How's this for a well-oiled propaganda machine? Long ago, vaccine manufacturers and public officials realized that the best way to sell their dangerous and ineffective vaccines to the public and medical professionals is to use . . . confusion. And has been working ever since. For example, most people don't know that 90 percent of the cases of HPV (human papilloma virus) infections clear up by themselves, and purported the link to cervical cancer isn't as clear cut as one might be led to believe. The virus needs decades to initiate cervical cancer — and the link is probably more closely associated with chronic inflammation of the cervix than the effect of the virus. This might explain why other viruses — and even bacterial infections — can also cause cervical cancer. A recent study found that women with the infection who have a high viral load (many viruses in their blood) can lower the risk of developing a cervical cancer condition 79 percent, if they take multivitamins. Incredibly, women with a low viral load who took multivitamins — vitamin A, E, or C — had a 65 percent lower risk of developing CIN 1, and an 89 percent lower risk of developing CIN 2 and CIN 3. And, they had almost no risk of ever developing cervical cancer. The authors of the study emphasized that having the infection alone did not increase a woman's risk of developing cervical cancer — each woman's nutritional status played a more important role. And since the Gardisal vaccine has already been responsible for a number of girls' deaths and seriously harmed thousands, we should be getting the word out for girls to choose multivitamins over death.

Worse Month for Army Suicides Remembered

This June marks the one year anniversary of the highest number of Army combatant suicides associated with the Iraq and Afghanistan war. I mention this grim date here in hopes of bringing it to as widespread attention as possible. There is a well-documented, strong connection between a fluorinated anti-malarial drug used by the Army, and these suicides, and has even been confirmed as a problem with elite Canadian troops. Still, the Pentagon continues to use the medication. But that's not all. There is evidence that the high number of vaccinations soldiers are required to get over a short period of time can trigger inflammation and immuno excitotoxicity in adults, and produce depression, which can ultimately lead to suicide when coupled with combat stress.

The Media thinks that nutrients are dangerous:

The Media and the Media elite certainly seem to think so, but what's the truth? According to a study in the annual report of the American Association of Poison Control Centers, (published in the journal *Clinical Toxicology*), there were no deaths from either vitamin or mineral supplements, ZERO. And, consider this: Several years ago, one study found about 100,000 deaths per year for pharmaceutical drugs and none for natural supplements, and, in a decade, pharmaceuticals kill one million people — that's more than all the American servicemen and women killed in World War I, World War II, Korea, Vietnam, and the Gulf War — combined! Meanwhile, despite this glaring disparity, the government and the medical elite are convinced we need to outlaw over-the counter natural supplements because "they're too dangerous." Have a look at Carolyn Dean's book, **Death by Modern Medicine**, for more information on the dangers of medical care.

Traditional Medicine
12 Cannot Stop
Atherosclerosis

L ow Vitamin D3 levels contribute enormously to the risk of having a heart attack or heart failure. Reports one 2008 study: from the slightly lowered to the lowest levels, men's risk of heart attacks increased 60 to 200 percent. **(Health Masters' Ultimate D3 5000)** After Bill Clinton's heart attack, he was treated with stent insertion, a small metal tube laced at the site of blocked coronary arteries. Since then, despite carefully following orthodox medical diet recommendation, exercising, and religiously taking his statin drugs, he's had several repeat surgeries to replace the stents, which are now blocked off with atherosclerotic buildup. What this means is that Clinton's atherosclerosis has progressed as if he had done nothing, which is actually a typical result for most coronary artery stent patients within three to five years of the surgery. Among the reasons why traditional medicine's prescriptions for atherosclerosis haven't worked:

- The stainless steel stents contain nickel, which can often stimulating immune reactions leading to atherosclerosis;
- The suggested "heart healthy diet" is alarmingly high in atherosclerosis-accelerating omega-6 fats;
- Dangerous and overrated statins don't work. In fact, every study shows they're no more effective than taking a daily aspirin.

Concerned about the health of your heart? Then call my office at 1-800-726-1834 and get on my Healthy Heart Program. I know it works because I take it every day. And by the way, statistically, a large number of nutraceuticals have proven that they can halt — or even reverse — the progression of atherosclerosis. That's why and how we put together our **Healthy Heart Program.**

Nutraceuticals that prevent atherosclerosis include the following:

- Ellagic acid (high in pomegranates)
- Curcumin
- Quercetin)
- Resveratrol (Health Masters' Resveratrol Plus)
- Natural vitamin E (Health Masters' Super Potent E)
- Vitamin C (Health Masters' Excellent C)
- Vitamin D3 (Health Masters' Ultimate D3 5000)
- Vitamin B12 (Health Masters' Sublingual B12)
- Vitamin B6 (Health Masters' Cortico B5 B6)
- Folate
- Magnesium (Health Masters' Magnesium Glycinate)
- Omega-3 oils (Health Masters' Norwegian Omega3)
- Garlic extract (Health Masters' Garlic).

This research examined the ability of the nutraceuticals to actually inhibit atherosclerosis by pathological examinations of the vessels themselves. Most statin research talks about "reducing risk factors," without looking at the blood vessel itself. Thanks, in part to a 2008 Health Professionals Study, in Arch Intern Med, we know that low vitamin D3 levels is a major connection to the risk of having a heart attack, coronary artery calcification, high blood pressure and heart failure. (Health Masters' Ultimate D3 5000) Men at the lowest levels of vitamin D3 levels were at risk of a heart attack over 200 percent, while men with a slightly lower level (near the recommend level of 30 ng/ml) had an increased heart attack risk of 60 percent. Vitamin D3 is thought to work by inhibiting atherosclerosis by reducing inflammation, inhibiting the reninangiotensin system (this is related to hypertension), suppressing foam cell formation, preventing cell proliferation in the heart and blood vessels and preventing lipid oxidation. Combining magnesium and vitamin D3 dramatically increases the vitamin's effectiveness.

Ask Dr. Ted:

Q: **After cancer, which is better for exercise: the treadmill or an elliptical machine?**

A: They're both good. It is also important to use light weights or a resistance machine as well, so that all muscles are exercised and enough resistance is used to strengthen the bones as well as muscles. And be careful not to overdo it as extreme exercise can produce immune suppression and excessive free radical generation.

Q: **I'm a vegan and I want to be certain of getting the proper amount of protein in my diet, any suggestions?**

A: That's easy: eat organic eggs. Eggs can replace the missing amino acids from a pure vegetarian diet: Egg whites contain a full and well-balanced complement to all the amino acids and egg yolks give you a full complement of phospholipids, the essential building blocks for cardiovascular and brain health. Just one caveat: don't scramble the eggs. Scrambling exposes them to air while cooking causes harmful oxidization of the lipids. And be sure to prepare your eggs in either extra-virgin olive oil or extra-virgin coconut oil. A dash or two of turmeric to the oil also reduces the risk of oxidizing the fats, and also tastes wonderful! If you have a problem eating eggs use my fit food protein. (Health Masters' Fit Food Protein). I use it every morning. It's fast, easy, and it tastes great.

Q: Is Splenda safe?

A: The short answer is this: NO! It's better to avoid this sweetener as a number of people have reported problems when using it. Research has also found, in addition to liver and kidney damage, intense skin reactions, damage to the thymus gland and immune impairment. Use Health Masters' Stevia! Here's why: Splenda — the commercial name of a sucralose-based artificial sweetener derived from sugar — belongs to a class of compounds called chlorocarbons. This class of highly reactive chemicals includes carbon tetrachloride and several pesticides. Like those other compounds, sucralose was shown to cause liver and kidney damage in animal testing. Chlorine is highly reactive in tissues when combined with carbon atoms. People who say Splenda is safe point out that salt also contain chlorine. Here's why that argument doesn't work: In excess, salt is extremely toxic to many tissues and, salt is not a chlorocarbons and is composed of sodium and chlorine.

Q: What do you suggest for controlling steadily progressing degenerative nerve disease?

A: Several things:

1. Have the test to diagnose gluten sensitivity — the tissue transglutaminase (tTG) and the anti-gliadin antibody test.
2. Have a full spectrum food allergy test as other food allergies can either cause the problem or worsen it.
3. Take the supplements which have shown to be beneficial, including: high-dose B1(Health Masters' B Complex), pyridoxal-5-phosphate, riboflavin(Health Masters' GHI Cleanse), 5-phosphate, moderate dose niacinamide (Health Masters' GHI Cleanse), natural (mixed) tocotrienols and tocopherols (Health Masters' Super Potent E), acetyl-L-Carnitine (Health Masters' Brain Focus), zinc (Health Masters' Zinc Glycinate), magnesium (Health Masters' Magnesium

Glycinate), selenium (Health Masters' E400 With Selenium), DHA (Health Masters' Norwegian Omega3) .

4. Avoid excitotoxin food additives (which plays a major role in neuropathy pain), inflammatory oils (corn, soybean, safflower, sunflower, peanut and canola oils), and extreme heat. Hot baths will make the condition significantly worse; cool baths will improve the symptoms.

5. Eat mainly vegetables and few meats, avoid breads which contain gluten, and drink white tea several times a day.

6. Avoid using insecticides indoors.

7. Stay away from all artificial dyes (especially yellow) as they can be very toxic and causes skin itching. I know, as I'm personally sensitive to it.

Q: Which supplements do you believe are effective in preventing cervical cancer?

A: Cervical cancer is a horrible disease for which there are nutraceuticals that can help to reduce the risk. Included in this list are a variety of supplements to help support the immune system. Please call my office at 1-800-726-1834 for details. Above all, I recommend combining dietary changes — like avoiding things known to promote cancer growth — and stimulating the immune system. Both of these things combined dramatically enhance the effectiveness of traditional cancer treatments while helping to prevent the disease. And of course, the most powerful anti-cancer supplements include: curcumin and quercetin (Health Masters' GHI Cleanse), ellagic acid (Health Masters' GHI Cleanse), DHA (Health Masters' Norwegian Omega3), hesperidin (Health Masters' Menopause Support), white and green tea extracts, and beta-glucan.

13 Is HEMMLA the New Miracle Product?

Rarely do I get really excited about the release of a new product. This time I am excited. My health is so good that I rarely feel a difference on new supplements. So when I hear about a new breakthrough I am always skeptical.

My response is always, " Okay, I will try it," but if I don't feel a difference in me, most of the time that's the end of the story. Well, guess what? I tried a new product several months ago and WOW!

In fact, I worked with Brian Blackburn, a biochemist that I know and we had some clinical studies done.

Here is what I personally experienced:

1. Immediate increase in Energy. (To the point of ridiculousness. I actually felt wired up for about 3 weeks.) This feeling like I was on 10 cups of coffee lasted for about 3 weeks. Then my energy normalized, but to a higher level than I have known for years

2. Within 2 days I had immediate increase in mental clarity, to the point that I felt like I was 18 years young again. It was also the second day that my vision became more sensitive to light. When I was 18 or so I was very sensitive to light especially sunlight. This was very interesting, as it was probably due to my eyes functioning better.

3. My Metabolism sped up. I could actually feel my body giving off heat. Remember I am 57 years young.

4. My "mood" became very calm and focused. I really loved this part, because little things and stressors just don't seem to bother me.

5. I have had a joint issue for several years with my left shoulder. It actually felt pretty good using the **Proprietary Joint Relief & Joint Rebuilding Formula** prior to taking Body Balance HEMMLA but I could never do flat bench fly's.

Flat bench fly's are my favorite chest exercise...And since I tore my rotator cuff some 15 years ago this exercise has always been uncomfortable for me to perform. Guess What??

Today in the gym I did 4 sets of flat bench fly's with NO pain... The only thing I am doing differently is taking the Body Balance HEMMLA. Plus my strength is going up and I am actually getting "pumped up" in the gym again that hasn't happened for years.

So what can I say beyond what I just said?

What's interesting is the compound astaxanthin is the primary ingredient in this product.

The problem with using other products containing astaxanthin is that they use chemical solvents like benzene along with other carcinogens to extract the astaxanthin. We use a patented CO_2 (carbon dioxide) process to naturally extract the astaxanthin.

I can honestly say the breakthrough and release of this product has really got me excited.

Here's what HEMMLA stands for.

H stands for hormone stabilization

E stands for a massive energy increase

M stands for metabolism increase

M stands for Mood and Brain improvement

L stands for a better lipid profile(that's the ratio of the hdl to the ldl)

A stands for antioxidant. This is an amazing antioxidant.

One more thing. If for any reason you aren't 100% satisfied with **Body Balance (HEMMLA)** within the first 30 days, just call my office and we will issue you an immediate credit. You do not even need to send this product back to me. That's how confident I am in this product.

Astaxanthin is probably the best antioxidant ever discovered. **PERIOD**.

Its ability to support so many aspects of your youth—from your heart to your brain—is downright remarkable.

"I Believe that this product may hold THE KEY TO LIFELONG YOUTH!" Like I said above, I really feel GREAT!

But there's only one form of astaxanthin out there that I would never recommend!

IT'S THE CO_2 PROCESSED PRODUCT.

Astaxanthin is naturally found in *tiny* microalgae in the ocean and fresh water sources. The problem is cracking through the microalgae.

One option is to use solvents and chemicals to break down the microalgae barriers and pull it out.

But you already know how I feel about chemicals in our diet.

My source doesn't use chemical and solvents to process the astaxanthin. My source uses a clever technique that utilizes CO_2. It's called *Super Critical CO_2 Extraction*.

The question is: What makes astaxanthin so amazing and effective? Why have dozens of studies been dedicated to discovering its power?? Why is the name popping up in nearly every media outlet from an afternoon talk show to respected medical journals?

It's because *astaxanthin* has a **special property**.

Most antioxidants are either *fat-soluble* or *water-soluble* and the difference determines where that antioxidant is able to travel in your body.

That's why some antioxidants are better for your eyes...others are better for your heart...some are able to travel right into your cells to help support your immune system.

Put this anti-aging miracle under a microscope and any scientist can see... it's made up of fat-soluble *and* water-soluble properties. That means...

Astaxanthin can go almost anywhere in your body!

Not only that...but this revolutionary ability allows it travel to areas of the body that many other antioxidants simply can't reach at all!

And just *what kind* of power is astaxanthin delivering to your body? It's already been shown to pack more of an antioxidant punch than...vitamin E, zeaxanthin, lutein, and beta-carotene...that is right—better than beta-carotene and lutein! And up until now—those were considered to be the primary antioxidants in anti-aging.

It has up to 500 TIMES the antioxidant power of vitamin E!

A 2003 study in mice showed it protected against wear and tear caused by exercise.

In a 2006 animal study, **it helped maintain healthy blood pressure levels!**

And imagine this—in a 2008 study this Antioxidant helped keep blood flowing freely in dogs.

Get the goods right to where your brain will use them!

This product actually has the ability to travel through the blood brain barrier!

And once inside—the support it can deliver to your brain is HUGE!

Once it's past the blood-brain barrier, it makes quick work of free radicals it comes across.

In one animal study—it lowered oxidative stress markers. And in yet another animal study where mice were given doses of astaxanthin equal to 10 mg for humans, it even supported memory health.

This is one of the few substances that can cross the blood brain barrier and in doing so means it has INCREDIBLE potential in the research of memory support and cognitive health. Blood levels of long chain n-3 fatty acids and the risk of sudden death

http://www.nejm.org/doi/full/10.1056/NEJMoa012918#t=articleTop

Astaxanthin: a novel potential treatment for oxidative stress and inflammation in cardiovascular disease.

http://www.ajconline.org/article/S0002-9149(08)00219-1/abstract

Krill oil significantly decreases 2-arachidonoylglycerol (Inflammation Signal) plasma levels in obese subjects.

http://www.nutritionandmetabolism.com/content/8/1/7

Novel phytonutrient contributors to antioxidant protection against cardiovascular disease

http://www.deepdyve.com/lp/elsevier/novel-phytonutrient-contributors-to-antioxidant-protection-against-1HlUwMZWFu

Krill Oil Lowers Plasma C-Reactive Protein

http://www.jacn.org/content/26/1/39.full

Krill Oil Supplement Markedly Reduces TNFα Protein and TNFα Expression in High Fat - Fed Mice

http://www.nutritionandmetabolism.com/content/8/1/51

14 | These Over-the-Counter Pain Killers Can Kill

There are so many side effects associated with *these* drugs including itching skin that I avoid them. We have an excellent program using three different products to control so many problems. Good old fashioned Health Masters' all natural, super high potency, **Organic Fermented Cod Liver Oil**, combined with our **Proprietary Joint Rebuilding Formula**, and **Proprietary Herbal Joint Relief Formula** are amazing for getting rid of aches and pains. I am in my 50's. I don't go a day without using them and the results are incredible!

Before I share with you about this amazing trilogy of natural pain relief products (below) it is imperative for you to understand from a technical perspective the terrible side effects found in many of the over-the-counter pain medicines that are probably in your medicine cabinet!

WHAT ARE COX2 (COX-2) INHIBITORS AND HOW DO THEY WORK?

To understand COX-2 (COX2) Inhibitors, you first have to understand COX-1 (COX1) and what its role in the body is. Regular NSAIDS (generally COX-1 and COX-2 Inhibitors) work by inhibiting the production of prostaglandins (PGs). Prostaglandins are fatty-acid derivatives located all over your body that are well known for their inflammation and immune response effects. However, they also have many different roles in the body. A scientific list would read as such: PG's are involved in as diverse normal processes as ovulation, blood clotting, renal function, wound healing, vasomotor tone, platelet aggregation, differentiation of immune cells, nerve growth, bone metabolism, and initiation of labor. Pretty essential to your body, wouldn't you say?

If you are familiar with the fact that when you are using drugs such as aspirin, your blood thins and you bruise easier, that is a "side effect" of the COX-1 inhibitor. In the above list, that would fall under the blood clotting category. Remember, COX-1 inhibitors work by inhibiting PG's. Due to the acidity of the stomach, the cells of your stomach are replaced very quickly, within a few days. One of the major roles of PG's is to keep the lining of the stomach intact, and when your PG system is disrupted (say by taking COX-1 drugs like many NSAIDS) stomach irritation, digestive tract problems and even intestinal or stomach bleeding and death could occur.

COX-2 inhibitors were discovered later, as a "healthier, more targeted" way of treating the inflammation — without the side effects. This makes sense as COX-2 is found more commonly in inflammatory and immune cells than COX-1 drugs, which exist throughout the body. Unfortunately, this would prove to be far, far from the truth. While COX-2 is more specific to inflammation, the side effects can be worse than COX-1 drugs.

NSAID Side Effects:

The side effects of COX-1 drugs are pretty terrible. It is estimated that 25% experience some kind of side effect and 5% develop SERIOUS health consequences such as GI (stomach) bleeding, acute renal failure, or worse.

The New England Journal of Medicine reports that "anti-inflammatory drugs (prescription and over-the-counter, which include Advil®, Motrin®, Aleve®, Ordus®, Aspirin, and over 20 others) alone cause over 16,500 deaths and over 103,000 hospitalizations per year in the US", according to a review article published in the New England Journal of Medicine [1].

You can see why researchers would believe there was a clear cut and dry line between COX-1 and COX-2. The message was clear: research (and get patents for) drugs that actually inhibited only COX-2 and you would have a blockbuster drug on your hands. Unfortunately, like many things, it was not nearly as cut and dry as this. Over the counter drugs such as Ibuprofen and Naproxen work to inhibit COX-1 and COX-2. Aspirin works more on COX-1. Some others such as diclofenac work primarily on COX-2 but also affect COX-1. However, even "selective" COX-2 inhibitors aren't that selective. At therapeutic dosages, they inhibit enough COX-1 to potentially cause the same stomach toxicity and other associated problems as COX-1. Not to the exact same extent, but more than enough to do damage.

Remember, 16,500 people are KILLED by "harmless" and "common" NSAIDS such as aspirin or ibuprofen every year. In development are other "newer aspirins" that may prove to ACTUALLY be more selective for COX-2 than COX-1, but in the mean time — despite claims of being "selective" —

the current COX-2's such as Vioxx® (rofecoxib) or (celecoxib) are simply not selective enough, not to mention some of their potentially horrible side effects and the associated lawsuits that have been filed due to side effects such as heart attacks, stroke and blood clots2. Our advice is to explore (for osteoarthritis) other alternative, cheaper and far more effective treatments for your pain. Glucosamine is a natural (and as such not patentable by large drug companies) substance that has been shown to not just be at least as effective as Ibuprofen and other related drugs but also can slow or maybe even stop the spread of osteoarthritis. Plus, it works to rejuvenate cartilage and rebuild the damage that has already occurred. Not even a pure "second generation" COX-2 drug will be able to do that.

References: 1. Wolfe MM, et. al. NEJM 1999;340(24):1888-99

Now some GOOD GREAT News!

We have finally developed a clinically tested natural pain management product combined with a new joint product that has been clinically proven to re-grow cartilage and naturally manage pain especially when used in conjunction with our good old fashioned Health Masters' all natural, super high potency, **Organic Fermented Cod Liver Oil**. Wow! What a breakthrough! We have named these two products Health Masters' **Proprietary Joint Rebuilding Formula**, and **Proprietary Herbal Joint Relief Formula**.

After 30 years in the nutraceutical and wellness business it has become increasingly more difficult to get me excited about new product releases. **Well, guess what? This one excites me!**

But, there is one thing I have got to tell you. You all know that I don't eat pork or shellfish but there are exceptions to products made from them. An example: thyroid extract from pork and insulin from pork. Both of these products have been real life savers. So when we started working on the joint product I was hesitant to use green mussel extract. In the initial research we did not want to include the extract. The problem is the results including it have been nothing short of miraculous. This product really works! So again, to me it falls into the categories of insulin and thyroid extract with the same incredible results. It is kind of like soy. I can't stand it and won't eat it but in some of our products the highest quality source of vitamin E is derived from soy. You know I tell you not to eat soy but the vitamin E from soy is great. That's the way the green mussel extract works. I don't eat shellfish nor would I ever willingly do so but I do use and endorse this product.

My mother- in- law is 78 years young. She loves the product and what it has done for her joints. My wife Sharon is an active 56 year young mother of four. We exercise together 6 days a week and both of us have experienced joint improvement using this product. It has literally been a miracle for my wife's joints. Many of you may not know this but my wife is a black belt in Karate. She even won the weapons competition in the US open which is a world martial arts competition. Well to be blunt, she really messed up her shoulders, elbows, and wrists during her years in martial arts. Guess what? These two products have completely gotten rid of all her joint pain. Combining these products with **HGH Stimulate** has literally turned back the hands of time. She has even started doing pull-ups. The other day while watching her do pull-ups, I reminded her that she was 56. She smiled and said, " I feel like I am 20 years old." Age is just a number. Then she continued doing more pull-ups. I must say God has really blessed me with an incredible wife. We have been married for 25 years. Twenty-four of those years have been great. As I have written before, one year was rough when she started menopause. But after we discovered a hormone stabilization program she was back to normal. It's exciting to me I have a wife who looks 30, works out like a teenager, is an incredible mother and wife, and who eats right and has written multiple bestselling books. Wow, I feel so blessed! Well, enough of all the mushy stuff. I must tell you it was my privilege to develop a product that has fixed her joints.

So here is my commitment to you: Use these two products for 90 days as directed. If you do not have the same incredible results that Sharon, myself, my mother in law, and the clinical trial participants have experienced, keep the product and I will give you a full credit in my office for the full purchase price of your order up to a three months' supply. Plus, you don't even need to return the unused portion. . You see, I have already run the clinical trials. I know the results that you're going to get. I can't make a better offer than a no-risk-trial.

Proprietary Herbal Joint Relief Formula

Relieves pain associated with arthritis and arthrosis, morning stiffness and low back pain.

Proprietary Joint Rebuilding Formula,

Helps protect and develop healthy cartilage, prevents pain associated to arthrosis and improves mobility and flexibility of articulations.

Organic Fermented Cod Liver Oil

Good old fashioned Health Masters' all natural, super high potency, Organic Fermented Cod Liver Oil.

References

1. Jang MH, et al. Harpagophytum procumbens suppresses lipopolysaccharide-stimulated expressions of cyclooxygenase-2 and inducible nitric oxide synthase in firbroblast cell line L929. J Pharmacol. Sci., 2003, 93(3): p. 367-371.

2. Loew D, et al. Investigation on the pharmacokinetic properties of Harpagophytum extracts and their effects on eicosanoid biosynthesis in vitro and ex vivo. Clin. Pharmacol. Ther., 2001. 69(5): p. 356-364.

3. Schulze-Tanzil G, et al. Effect of a Harpagophytum procumbens DC extract on matrix metalloproteinases in human chondrocytes in vitro. Arzneimittelforschung, 2004. 54(4): p.213-220

4. Litlle C, Parsons T. Herbal therapy for treating rheumatoid arthritis. Cochrane Database Syst. Rev. 2001: (1) : CD002948

5. Garbacki N, et al. Effects of prodelphinidins isolated from Ribes nigrum on chondrocyte metabolism and COX activity. Naunyn Schmiedebergs Arch Pharmacol. 2002 Jun;365(6):434-41. Epub 2002 Apr 26

6. Miller T, Wu H. In vivo evidence for prostaglandin inhibitory activity in New Zealand green-lipped mussel extract. N Z Med J. 1984 Jun 13;97(757):355-7.

7. Curtis CL, et al. Pathologic indicators of degradation and inflammation in human osteoarthritic cartilage are abrogated by exposure to n-3 fatty acids., Arthritis Rheum. 2002 Jun;46(6):1544-53.

8. Curtis CL, et al. n-3 fatty acids specifically modulate catabolic factors involved in articular cartilage degradation., J Biol Chem. 2000 Jan 14;275(2):721-4

9. S.L.M. Gibson and R.G. Gibson. The treatment of arthritis with a lipid extract of Perna canaliculus: a randomized trial. Complement Ther Med 1998;6:122-6.

10. LAU CS et al. Treatment of knee osteoarthritis with Lyprinol®, lipid extract of the green-lipped mussel – a doubleblind placebo-controlled study. Progress in Nutrition 2004; 6(1):17-31.

11. Cho SH, et al. Clinical efficacy and safety of Lyprinol, a patented extract from New Zealand green-lipped mussel (Perna Canaliculus) in patients with osteoarthritis of the hip and knee: Multicenter Clinical Trial with a 2-months treatment period. The Newest Medical Journal 2002; 45(5):27-33.

12. Chrubasik S, Eisenberg E, et al. Treatment of low back pain exacerbations with willow bark extract: a randomized double-blind study. Am J Med 2000 Jul;109(1):9-14.

13. Chrubasik S, Kunzel O, et al. Treatment of low back pain with a herbal or synthetic anti-rheumatic: a randomized controlled study. Willow bark extract for low back pain. Rheumatology (Oxford). 2001 Dec;40(12):1388-93.

14. Schmid B, Ludtke R, et al. Efficacy and tolerability of a standardized willow bark extract in patients with osteoarthritis: randomized placebo-controlled, double blind clinical trial. Phytother Res 2001 Jun;15(4):344-50.

15. Fiebich BL, Chrubasik S. Effects of an ethanolic salix extract on the release of selected inflammatory mediators in vitro., Phytomedicine. 2004 Feb;11(2-3):135-8.

16. Smolinski AT, Pestka JJ. Comparative effects of the herbal constituent parthenolide (Feverfew) on lipopolysaccharide-induced inflammatory gene expression in murine spleen and liver. J Inflamm (Lond). 2005 Jun 29;2:6.

17. Calliste CA, Trouillas P, Allais DP, Simon A, Duroux JL, Free radical scavenging activities measured by electron spin resonance spectroscopy and B16 cell antiproliferative behaviors of seven plants., J Agric Food Chem. 2001 Jul;49(7):3321-7.

18. Evidence-based Systematic Review of Birch by the Natural Standard Research Collaboration. Copyright ® 2007. www.naturalstandard.coma>. Accessed 12/12/2008.

19. Peter Holmes, Birch Leaf and Bark. In: The Energetics of Western Herbs: A Materia Medica Integrating Western & Chinese Herbal Therapies. Page 705, Volume 2. Fourth edition, 2006. South Lotus Press.

Caution: Consult a healthcare practitioner before using this product if you are pregnant or breastfeeding, taking a blood thinner, if you are taking anti-arrhythmic medication or if you have or suspect you have any other medical condition or are taking any prescription drugs. Avoid if sensitive to salicylates. Do not exceed the recommended daily intake. Do not use if security seal is broken. Keep out of reach of children. Store at room temperature.

PROPRIETARY JOINT REBUILDING FORMULA

Proprietary Joint Rebuilding Formula, a member of **Health Masters' Exclusive and Patented ("EP")** line is the result of Health Masters' partnership with Biotanika™, a Canadian company that develops evidence-based natural health products for pain management. It is among a group of formulas that also includes **Proprietary Joint Rebuilding Formula** . The formulation of it began with researchers at Biotanika investigating the potential of traditional herb extracts to act additively or synergistically to reduce inflammation and pain using the lowest doses of each herb. Biotanika used three pre-clinical test protocols that are recognized by the scientific community as good models for inflammatory diseases. These tests resulted in formulas benchmarked with current standards of care used in western medicine.

The primary goal of the first clinical trial of the two formulas was to assess the safety and efficacy for the relief of pain in fourteen patients with either low back pain, joint (knee, shoulder, or hip) pain, or muscular or articular pain (the majority had moderate-to-severe pain). These patients had visited a natural health care practitioner seeking alternative therapies to NSAIDs or surgery. As is most often seen in patients scheduled for knee replacement surgery or who have had knee replacements, benefit was nil. However, all patients with low back, hip and shoulder pain demonstrated significant benefit.

- **Glucosamine Sulfate**, a chondro-protective agent occurring naturally in all human tissues, appears to stimulate the manufacture of cartilage components and the deposition of sulfur into the cartilage. In combination with chondroitin sulfate it may be effective in patients with moderate-to-severe knee pain [1,2,3].

- **Methylsulfonylmethane** (MSM) is a naturally-occurring, sulfur-containing, water-soluble compound (AKA DMSO2) has been demonstrated to possess anti-inflammatory and antioxidant properties [4,5].

- **Chondroitin Sulfate**, a primary proteoglycan in the body, attracts and retains a significant quantity of water guaranteeing cartilage resistance and elasticity. It has anti-inflammatory and antioxidative properties. [7,8].

- **Hyaluronic Acid**, a naturally occurring glycosaminoglycan in synovial fluid, helps create a viscous environment, cushion joints and maintains normal joint function. It has anti-inflammatory and antioxidant properties [9,10]

- **Vitamin C and Manganese** — Vitamin C is essential for synthesis of collagen and for maintaining its integrity. Manganese is important in the growth and development of normal bone and in the synthesis of cartilage [11]. Studies in rats, rabbits and humans have demonstrated a joint supportive, anti-inflammatory effect of a combination of glucosamine, chondroitin and manganese ascorbate. [21,22].

References

1. Distler J, Anguelouch A. Evidence-based practice: review of clinical evidence on the efficacy of glucosamine and chondroitin in the treatment of osteoarthritis. J Am Acad Nurse Pract. 2006 Oct;18(10):487-93 [PMID: 16999714]
2. Clegg DO, et al. Glucosamine, chondroitin sulfate, and the two in combination for painful knee osteoarthritis. N Engl J Med. 2006 Feb 23;354(8):795-808 [PMID: 16495392]
3. Matheson AJ, Perry CM. Glucosamine: a review of its use in the management of osteoarthritis. Drugs Aging. 2003;20(14):1041-60 [PMID:14651444]
4. Parcell S. Sulfur in human nutrition and applications in medicine. Altern Med Rev. 2002 Feb;7(1):22-44 [PMID: 11896744]
5. Beilke MA, et al. Effects of dimethyl sulfoxide on the oxidative function of human neutrophils. J Lab Clin Med 1987, 110:91-96 [PMID:3598341]
7. Chan PS. Glucosamine and chondroitin sulfate regulate gene expression and synthesis of nitric oxide and prostaglandin E(2) in articular cartilage explants. Osteoarthritis Cartilage. 2005 May;13(5):387-94 [PMID: 15882562]
8. Ha BJ. Oxidative stress in ovariectomy menopause and role of chondroitin sulfate. Arch Pharm Res. 2004 Aug;27(8):867-72 [PMID: 15460450]
9. Campo GM, et al. Aromatic trap analysis of free radicals production in experimental collagen-induced arthritis in the rat: protective effect of glycosaminoglycans treatment. Free Radic Res. 2003 Mar;37(3):257-68.[PMID: 12688421]
10. Campo GM, et al. Administration of hyaluronic acid and chondroitin-4-sulfate limits endogenous antioxidant depletion and reduces cell damage in experimental acute pancreatitis. Pancreas. 2004 Mar;28(2):E45-53. [PMID: 15028960]
11. Strause L, et al.The effect of deficiencies of manganese and copper on osteoinduction and on resorption of bone particles in rats. Calcif Tissue Int. 1987 Sep;41(3):145-50. [PMID: 3117341]
12. Beren J, et al. Effect of pre-loading oral glucosamine HCl/chondroitin sulfate/manganese ascorbate combination on experimental arthritis in rats. Exp Biol Med (Maywood). 2001 Feb;226(2):144-51 [PMID:11446439]
13. Das A Jr, et al. Efficacy of a combination of FCHG49 glucosamine hydrochloride, TRH122 low molecular weight sodium chondroitin sulfate and manganese ascorbate in the management of knee osteoarthritis. Osteoarthritis Cartilage.

CHONDROCYTES: CRITICAL CELLS FOR THE HEALTH OF OUR CARTILAGE

Chondrocytes are key cells in our cartilage. It produces and maintains the cartilage tissue, that consists essentially of collagen and proteoglycan. They are essential for the regeneration of the cartilage.

Proprietary Herbal Joint Relief Formula and **Proprietary Joint Rebuilding Formula** outperform glucosamine and chondroitin.

Microscopic look at the articulation with osteoarthritis (histochemical analysis of the tissues).

Inflammation is the "initiator" of many discomforts

Many preclinical studies have been performed. These studies demonstrated that the combination of Proprietary Herbal Joint Relief Formula and Proprietary Joint Rebuilding Formula modulates certain intermediates responsible for inflammation thereby reducing the swelling and associated pain.

Finally, a natural medicine line of natural health products!

- Ingredients were selected based on independent scientific research that demonstrated their safety and efficacy.
- Products tested in preclinical models used by the pharmaceutical industry.
- A rigorous quality control program: each batch of ingredients and final product is tested by an independent laboratory to assure that it conforms to specifications (purity, identity) and that it is free of contaminants or adulterants such as heavy metals, pesticides, synthetic NSAIDs. Testing program includes confirming plant part and subspecies.
- Management team consists of professionals from the pharmaceutical industry and 25 years of nutraceutical research.
- Solid experience in preclinical and clinical product development as well as regulatory affairs and natural health products.

Scientific Facts

- **Arthritis:** a chronic degenerative disease of the articulations (cartilage); its evolution limits the mobility of the articulations and causes pain, swelling and loss of joint flexibility.
- **Arthrosis:** is the most frequent form of arthritis; a disease associated with stress/injury to the articulations; it progresses in acute phases; often associated with age or old accidents/injuries to the articulations.
- **Advancements:** better understanding of the mechanisms involved in the degeneration of cartilage and the development of alternative treatments that are less damaging to the GI tract.
- **Benefits:** improvement in the quality of life such as better joint flexibility and mobility and reduced pain.

15 | Doing This May Cause You to Die in Your Sleep

Sadly, folks don't realize how dangerous sleeping pills really are! I will tell you the truth about their death rates and how to sleep like a baby without them. Quite frankly, I have never been a fan of games of chance. Russian roulette has never nor never will it be something that could possibly interest me. The problem is, many folks are playing that game at night when they take a sleeping pill. One night you may not wake up again. Isn't that special?

New numbers show that sleeping pills swallowed by millions every night could be linked to up to 500,000 deaths a year. This number is so insanely high that it would actually be the number three cause of death in the entire country, right behind heart disease and cancer . Here are some of the statistics: 35,000 people were actually tracked for 2.5 years. Here is what was learned. If you take 132 sleeping pills a year, you are 5.3 times as likely to die as non-users. But, that is only the beginning!

Some pills actually pack even more of a deadly punch. The heaviest users of Zolpidem (aka Ambien) boosts the risk up to 5.7 times death and temazepam (aka Restoril) raises the risk to 6.6 times death. By the way, these statistics come from the British Medical Journal. And since I seem to be the bearer of unpleasant information, I might as well give you another interesting tidbit: heavy sleeping pill users also have a 35% greater chance of cancer. This is why I think this cancer rate increases.

Remember when many of you first heard me tell you that 3 hot-dogs a week eaten by a child increased the rate of leukemia by 12 times...I have a news flash for you: it is not just the hot-dogs...it's the lifestyle that many children have due to their parents. Okay, don't get mad at me over this one, but I have never seen a two year old drive to the store to buy junk food. So the reality is, if you are drinking and smoking and eating junk food all day and sucking down coffee you aren't going to sleep well at night, and if you indoctrinate your children into this lifestyle, they have a very high probability of getting cancer, heart disease and diabetes.

So, please eat right and please teach your kids to do the same. Sorry about the Segway, but I really believe this info is critical . The reality is if you take the sleeping pills to sleep you are simply masking the symptoms of why you cannot sleep. Does that make sense to you? You don't have a deficiency of sleeping pills! Well, it does make sense to me...and I sleep great at night and I am 56 years young! But, I will tell you what Sharon and I do in a minute. Don't think you can rest easy if you're not a big-time sleeping pill popper. The same study finds that people who took just 18 pills or fewer a year, more than tripled their death risk... and more than 18 a year more than quadrupled it. Now that one even surprised me. But the reality is many of these statistics are caused again by the lifestyle choices we all make.

Finally, there is one more topic I want to point out which deals with the lack of mental acuity and behavioral changes that occurs with sleeping pills. But this time I want you involved in this research, so I want you to Google the deadly side effects, loss of mental acuity, death rates, suicide and bizarre behavior of Ambien and Restoril, then make you own decision about these products.

So, let's get to the answer on how to sleep like a baby every night. One of the primary causes of sleepless nights can be as simple as a calcium deficiency! Remember what your grandmother used to say: "a glass of warm milk before bed." But, make sure the milk is organic and NON Homogenized...that's really important. Don't ever drink homogenized milk. If you are over 50, you can remember how the milk used to separate? The milk fat would literally, after a few days, float to the top of the glass container. Well, that is what milk is supposed to do. If you live in a state that you can still buy raw certified organic milk, that's the best. Women, the easiest way to get calcium if you don't like milk, is to eat organic yogurt as an alternative for calcium or you can take one of our incredible calcium supplements. Either way women need more calcium than men.

Men, I don't take calcium supplements nor do I recommend you do unless you are trying to correct a pH imbalance. I use a cup of the organic non-homogenized milk every morning for my calcium needs which I mix with the **Fit Food**. Secondly, one hour before bedtime I also take our **Enhanced Sleep Support** along with a **Melatonin Sublingual**. I swallow the sleep support and chew the Melatonin and let it dissolve under my tongue. The **Enhanced Sleep Support** helps to reduce cortisol which keeps you awake while the **Melatonin** is a natural product produced by the pineal gland. Our natural production of Melatonin decreases past the age of 40. This combination lets me sleep like a baby every night. This is the best natural approach to a great night's sleep my wife and I have found.

16 Vitamin Deficiency Can Cause Confusion, Fatigue, Dementia

Deficiencies can cause a wide variety of symptoms. These symptoms can quickly be misdiagnosed as disease. The disease is then treated instead of the deficiency. As the deficiency gets worse, the symptoms are drugged and seem to go away. The person then believes they have gotten better. Over a period of time the medication no longer covers up the symptoms and stronger medication is used. If that medication doesn't work in most cases more advanced treatment is used including surgery. Back in the 50's when people had certain vitamin deficiencies which resulted in hypoglycemia, violent or aggressive behavior, lobotomies and electro-convulsive shock treatment were used.

Here's the irony: In most cases dietary change and supplementation could have corrected the deficiency causing the symptoms. The use of prescription drugs especially in the field of Psychiatry has become ridiculous.

"Dr. Weston A. Price, a researcher in the 1930's found that primitive tribes eating a whole foods, natural diet high in animal foods and animal fat had no need for prisons. The moral character of these isolated people was strong. They were not incapacitated mentally or physically..."

One nutritional deficiency in particular that may have the potential to wreak havoc on your psyche is niacin (vitamin B3). Pellagra is a condition caused by niacin deficiency, and is clinically manifested by the 4 D's:

1. Photosensitive dermatitis
2. Diarrhea
3. Dementia, and
4. Death

Pellagra's Vitamin B3
Deficiency Violent Side Effects:

A key point Dr. Saul brings up is that certain people have what Dr. Hoffer referred to as niacin dependency, meaning they need more niacin on a regular basis. Essentially, they're beyond deficient—they're dependent on high-doses of niacin in order to remain well. This particularly appears to be the case with mental disorders.

"Dr. Hoffer said that drug therapy alone has a cure rate of 10 percent. He added to that, The disease originates in your gut, with GI tract symptoms preceding dermatitis, and the condition is well known to be associated with undernourishment and the "poor man's diet" consisting primarily of corn products. Pellagra was epidemic in the American South during the early 1900's, and we just might be dealing with a similar epidemic of malnutrition today. A quote from the book, *Nourishing Traditions*: The Cookbook that Challenges Politically Correct Nutrition and the Diet Dictocrats read:

"The clinical description of the typical poor Southerner, any time between about 1900 and 1940, comes alive in the novels of William Faulkner—the brooding sullenness, suddenly shattered by outbursts of irrational anger, persecution, mania, the feeling of people living in a cruel and demented world of their own…Doctors knew very well that diet was at the bottom of all the misery they saw around them, and that disease could be kept at bay by a balanced food supply…"

While this deficiency may have caused some of these problems, there are other factors to consider. The Civil War was still very much alive in the memories of the south in the early 1900's. Many Grandfathers and Great Grandfathers were still alive and very angry at what had transpired with the Civil War. There is also the factor that the anger from these family members was part of the attitudes of the Grandchildren and relatives. I still remember in 1960 when I started school as a 1st grader many of the other students still hated "Yankees". There are homes in the South that still fly the Confederate Flag to this day.

Hartke continues:

"… Barbara Stitt, an author who once worked as a probation officer… found that changing the diet of ex-offenders eliminated the hostility and other symptoms that would lead them to act out in a criminal fashion. Her book is aptly titled, *Food & Behavior: A Natural Connection* and her work seems to confirm the findings of Dr. Weston A. Price on nutritional injury and the role it plays in juvenile delinquency and adult crimes.

A review of Barbara's book mentions her concern about reactive hypoglycemia, sub-clinical pellegra and vitamin B deficiencies being at the root of violent criminal's actions. Check out this revealing quote from the review: "The startling part of sub-clinical pellagra, like hypoglycemia, is that the symptoms also mirror those of schizophrenia, a problem so widespread that those who suffer from it occupy one out of every four hospital beds in the United States."

Dr. Stitt's book also discusses other vitamin B deficiencies, such as B1, B2, B6 and B12—all of which have an uncanny ability to produce symptoms of neuropsychiatric disorders.

Niacin for Schizophrenia?

Hoffer and Saul who are quoted below are two experts in the field of niacin usage:

Niacin, Dr. Hoffer found, may indeed be a "secret" treatment for psychological disorders, including schizophrenia, which can be notoriously difficult to address.

"Dr. Hoffer is probably the world authority on therapeutic use of niacin. He started doing tests, studies, and research into niacin back in the early 1950's. And by 1954, Abram Hoffer had performed the first double-blind, placebo-controlled nutrition studies in the history of psychiatry," Dr. Andrew Saul says.

"Now, the early 50's were an odd time. Drugs were on the move; more were coming along. But they hadn't developed to the point where they are today, to put it mildly." Dr. Hoffer had a PhD in biochemistry, and he specialized in cereal biochemistry, which means the study of the vitamins and nutrients in grain. He was also a medical doctor. He was also a board-certified psychiatrist, and head of psychiatric research for one of the provinces in Canada... Dr. Hoffer observed that schizophrenia had symptoms that were very similar to those of pellagra.

Pellagra is extreme or total niacin deficiency. Pellagrins, also — in addition to skin problems and many other things — have mental illness symptoms.

When vitamin B3 or niacin was first added as an enrichment or as a fortification to flour, about half of the people in mental institutions went home. This is not a well-known fact. They were there not because they were mentally ill — because of genetic, environment, or social reasons — but because they were malnourished... He wondered about the half that didn't go home.

What about the people that had a little bit of niacin, but didn't get better? ... He started giving what at the time were preposterously **high doses of niacin: 3,000 milligrams a day. And he was curing schizophrenia in 80 percent of the cases.**

This is astonishing. The cure rate for schizophrenia with drug therapy is not particularly good. Dr. Hoffer saw again and again that niacin worked. Then he studied it, did the placebo-controlled, double-blind test, and started writing paper after paper on this. At that point, the American Psychiatric Association literally blacklisted him."

According to Dr. Saul, other researchers have since confirmed Dr. Hoffer's findings, and found that niacin can also be successfully used in the treatment of other mental disorders, such as:

- Attention deficit disorder
- General psychosis
- Anxiety
- Depression
- Obsessive-compulsive disorder
- Bipolar disorder

Can Anger and Behavioral Issues be "Miraculously" Solved with High-Dose Vitamin B3?

Here's another example From Dr. Saul for using niacin in the treatment of behavioral problems:

"I knew a neighbor who had a boy who was really, really in trouble — constantly in trouble at school, constantly in trouble at home. He was violent. This was really serious. This was more than ADHD. I'm calling it ADHD, because that's what the boy's doctors called it. But the fact is, it was far beyond that. Nevertheless, they gave him one of the usual drugs for Attention Deficit Disorder, and it made him worse."

So now he was even more violent and even more psychotic. The parents were in a state, as you can imagine, because the kid's only thirteen, and everything is falling apart at home. They learned about Dr. Hoffer's niacin approach. And because it was a child, they figured, "Well, we'll start him at a lower level." They gave him 1,500 milligrams a day of niacinamide.

Now, niacinamide and niacin have the same psychiatric benefits. They both work. The difference is niacin will cause a flush in almost everyone who takes it in quantity, especially for the first couple of weeks...

... The parents noticed an immediate improvement. Within days, the child was less angry. He was less troubled at school. He was less oppositional. He was less violent. They immediately figured that if a little helped, maybe more would help more. They wouldn't know unless they tried, and they had no other options. Again, medication was making him worse not better.

They took him totally off of his medication, and they increased his niacin to ultimately about 5,000 milligrams a day. They even got the boy's psychiatrist to prescribe niacin, so he could take it at school. The school nurse was giving the boy niacinamide twice a day at school, as well as at home. All of a sudden, calls were coming from the teachers, saying, "The kid was just transformed. He was doing great." At home, everything was better.

This young teenager was taking nearly 5,000 milligrams a day of Niacinamide. Now, this is an important caution for people thinking of doing this. Niacinamide has a disadvantage, and that is it's more likely to cause nausea at very high doses. And the boy did start experiencing nausea at around 5,000 milligrams a day. So, what they did was cut back the niacinamide quantity and started giving him more niacin. He got used to the flush. Then he was able to take the full high dose."

(I do not recommend this high dosage to anyone unless prescribed by a medical doctor trained in this field and monitored by blood and liver testing.)

How can drugs make a well person sick? How can drugs make a sick person well? " He saw this over and over and over and over again... Dr. Hoffer's experience was buttressed by Dr. Humphrey Osmond and a number of other researchers who have confirmed in practice that niacin is the best therapy for many forms of mental illness. And not only that, drug therapy is making people worse...

People would be better off — in many forms of mental illness — if they had no medication. But with niacin, we're not just negating, we're affirming. Niacin is a way that the person can tell within a few hours if it's going to help. If someone has anxiety, depression, psychosis, or schizophrenia, if they take high doses of niacin, they'll notice two things right away. The first: they're going to flush like crazy. And the second: they're going to feel better.

Now, as far as the "flush like crazy" thing goes, people are more concerned with the niacin flush than they need to be. But if you just can't contain the idea of having a niacin flush, take inositol hexaniacinate, and that will work just fine. Dr. Hoffer said, "The best cure for the niacin flush is more niacin." If you keep taking the niacin, the histamine flushes out of the body and the vasodilation stops. It takes, perhaps, a couple of weeks."

Can Vitamin B3 also be used to strengthen the body's immune system?

Research also suggests vitamin B3 may be able to combat superbugs that modern medicine is finding it harder to fight, including antibiotic-resistance staph infections. Research showed that high doses of the vitamin boosted the immune system by 1,000 times, giving the researchers hope that they may have found a new—and possibly better—way to fight infection.

According to BBC News

"B3 increases the numbers and efficacy of neutrophils, white blood cells that can kill and eat harmful bugs. The study, in the Journal of Clinical Investigation, could lead to a "major change in treatment", a UK expert said."

One of the researchers is quoted as saying:

"This could give us a new way to treat Staph infections that can be deadly, and might be used in combination with current antibiotics. It's a way to tap into the power of the innate immune system and stimulate it to provide a more powerful and natural immune response."

What does this all Mean?

Well, here's the bottom line. Years ago I wrote a book on Attention Deficit Disorder. The book is called *Maximum Solutions to ADD Autism and Learning Disabilities*. The book was written about ten years ago, but it is still excellent.

The primary theme of the book is that in many cases deficiencies and toxins can cause all types of behavioral problems.

When I wrote the book this actually was cutting edge controversial information.

The importance of B vitamins and essential fats for behavioral issues is repeatedly stated in my book.

So here's an updated guideline of supplements, based on current research:

- Ultimate Multiple
- B complex
- Corticare B5B6
- Vascular relaxant niacin
- Cod liver oil
- Living fuel
- Excellent C
- GHI cleanse
- D3-5000

17 | Do not use this Death Sweetener!

Almost 20 years ago I was contacted by the maker of aspartame to stop speaking badly about their product...I didn't stop! Now the whole world who reads, cares about their health and is educated, no longer drinks or eats products made with aspartame or Equal also known as NutraSweet. It causes brain cancer, memory loss and blindness. This list of side effects goes on and on.

But this is not about aspartame, it's about Sucralose also known as " Splenda."

Before I get started I need to share with you some of my observations.

Why is it that the FDA suppresses the use of vitamins and their research?

Why is it that the FDA allows poisonous drugs like Statins to be on the market?

Why is it that the FDA, EPA and other government agencies have turned a blind eye to the globalists doing global atmospheric engineering using aluminum, barium and strontium as reflective agents being sprayed into the atmosphere to supposedly combat global warming?

By the way I had my rain water tested twice. (I know you read this earlier, but it is worth repeating.) It contains barium and aluminum. Rain water is supposed to be pure like distilled water. The only way minerals are present in rainwater is if they have been placed in the air. There are several ways this can happen: volcanic eruptions, dust storms, industrial smoke stacks and aerosol dispersal.

Research has clearly shown that aluminum is implicated in Alzheimer's disease and that barium weakens the immune system. We inhale these products through our lungs, and into our bloodstreams. Plus these mineral compounds also alkalinize the soil causing massive crop reductions and crop failure. The only way that I know to remove them from your body is through the use of EDTA. We carry a product called **Chelation Therapy** which contains EDTA.

These types of questions have always intrigued me. It seems that in many cases the very government that we have hired to protect us is causing a lot of problems with our health. I realize that humans can make a lot of mistakes and that none of us are perfect , but this blatant disregard for the health and safety of humans around the globe is especially troubling to me.

Back to the subject:

What is " Splenda?"

Basically it is bug spray. You would just as soon put a pesticide in your food as Sucralose. Because Sucralose (Splenda) is a chlorocarbon (Pesticides are chlorocarbons) . Chlorocarbons have long been shown to cause organ, genetic, and reproductive damage. It should be no surprise, therefore, that the testing of Sucralose reveals that it can cause up to 40 percent shrinkage of the thymus: a gland that is the very foundation of our immune system.

Sucralose also causes swelling of the liver and kidneys, and CALCIFICATION of the kidney. Note: if you experience kidney pain, cramping, or an irritated bladder after using any Sucralose, stop use immediately. Sucralose is not sugar, it is not found in nature, it is toxic to humans just like bug spray.

Has Testing on lab animals shown it to be safe?

Testing that has been paid for by the manufacturer claims safety...Again, read my article I have previously written on aspartame, which you can find on our Healthmasters. Com web site. It has been shown over and over again that only independent testing with no financial ties produce accurate testing. I know of no such studies on Splenda. The independent studies that I have seen clearly implicate it in a variety of diseases.

Do any tests show Splenda causes cancer?

An animal that ingests chlorine (especially on a regular basis) is at risk of cancer. The *Merck Manuel* and *OSHA 40 SARA 120 Hazardous Waste Handbook* states that chlorine is a carcinogen and emergency procedures should be taken when exposed via swallowing, inhaling, or through the skin.

I personally believe potential cancers using Splenda are based upon how much you use and how often, your present and past health status, and the degree of other toxins you are putting into your body.

Good luck with that one ...I personally believe that this product is so toxic and will cause so many health problems that it's a toss- up whether the cancer it may cause will kill you before kidney calcification occurs and you die from kidney failure.

Let me ask you two more questions. How much pesticide does it take to kill you?

Do you really want know how much pesticide it takes to kills you?

If you want an alternative to artificial poisons used as sweeteners, please use Stevia.

We carry a brand at **www.healthmasters.com** that has NO aftertaste. It's inexpensive and it goes a long way.

In fact Sharon has learned to use it in baking. This is an incredible product.

And for those looking for a quality protein powder our **Fit Food whey protein** is also sweetened with stevia.

Here are some additional side effects that have been reported after Splenda usage:

- Enlarged liver and kidneys
- Atrophy of lymph follicles in the spleen and thymus
- Increased fecal weight
- Reduced growth rate
- Decreased red blood cell count
- Hyperplasia of the pelvis
- Extension of the pregnancy period
- Aborted pregnancy
- Decreased fetal body weights and placental weights
- Diarrhea
- Shrunken thymus glands (up to 40 percent shrinkage)

18

Stimulates Kill! How to feel great without them!

For the past few years, people have been seriously buying into the buzz over coffee and caffeinated energy drinks such as Red Bull™ as the best possible way to combat fatigue, lethargy and low energy. Red Bull™ is the most popular energy drink in the world and caffeine is its chief ingredient. With sales of all energy drinks expected to top $9 billion this year, is it any surprise that these drinks are the fastest growing segment of the U.S. beverage market? Sure, everyone needs a pick-me-up occasionally. Even I occasionally use a **Purple Stick Acai-Natural Energy Boost** in the morning before I work out. The difference here is that this product is a green tea extract and doesn't drain the adrenals or elevate cortisol levels.

The problem is, as a society, we're working harder and longer and in many cases, commuting further on a daily basis. So it's convenient to grab something to help us not feel wiped out by 11:00 AM . . . or completely drained by 3:00 PM . . . or ready to fall asleep behind the wheel on the drive home or to the gym. But, think about this: Are the side effects from those so-called energy drinks worth it? I'm talking about after consuming all that caffeine throughout the day, you're still awake at midnight — and if you do fall asleep, you just can't get the refreshing non-rapid eye movement sleep we all need. And guess what? Now you're tired all the time. And I haven't even mentioned the dangerous side effects of caffeine, like elevated heart rates, uncontrolled anxiety, depression, nausea and vomiting, restlessness, tremors and increased urination.

I think you get the point : Caffeinated beverages, energy drinks, and artificial stimulants — they're all bad! Now that you know this, you can begin to take care of your bodies by putting those so-called fast energy drinks and double mocha espresso shots with whipped cream where they belong — in the trash. What I'm going to do now is share with you the reason — the real reason — you're feeling so lethargic, so often. And then I'll also share with you the solution to that low energy crisis of yours that I trust and use. And in time, the only use you'll have for coffee grounds is to flavor a chocolate cake.

Why You Feel So Rundown So Often: The 21st century energy crisis isn't just at the pump . . . it's within you! Does this sound familiar? You're always on the run. Everything seems a whole lot harder for you than it should be. It's increasingly difficult to get out of bed in the morning. You depend on caffeine or sugar to bolster your flagging energy in the afternoon. You're feeling weary and irritable much of the time. You often crave salty foods or binge on sugar. You fall asleep while reading or while watching movies. You struggle to "come down" at night so you can get to sleep. If it does sound familiar to you, what I'm going to introduce you to will help restore your energy and balance your adrenal output (I'll explain this one in just a bit) so you can feel like yourself again. Those caffeinated beverage commercials and ads might poke fun at your 'low energy crisis', but the condition is nothing to laugh at.

There is a rather serious cause behind it — something which needs to be addressed by millions of Americans... RIGHT NOW! And the unfortunate thing is, all of us are under so much stress, that we tend to overlook the symptoms and warning signs of this condition. In fact, you know when something 'wrong' is done so often that it starts to feel 'normal.' That's what's happening here. We think nothing of pumping our bodies with quick, artificial stimulants to rev up our nervous system. And pretty soon we're so wired, we can't calm down. So what happens next? We overeat to relax . . . we drink . . . we smoke . . .we take tranquilizers and sleeping pills. And then wake up the next morning just to start the cycle of destruction all over again. I understand exactly what so many of you are going through. Many of you would be shocked to learn that when I was in graduate school at Florida State University, I was drinking 18 cups of coffee a day. Was I ever addicted! And to be perfectly honest with you, (which I always am!) it was really hard for me to stop and get off the coffee bandwagon. It wasn't until I was 27 years old and diagnosed with heart disease, that I finally realized that the coffee had to go! What I did to stop was gradually reduce the amount of caffeine I was ingesting over a three week period. It was tough. Still is — I love the way fresh brewed coffee smells. But I know how horrible I'll end up feeling if I have a cup, so I just avoid it altogether. Of course, I can hear some of you saying, "Why not switch to decaf?" Well, here's why not: the primary way coffee is decaffeinated is by soaking the coffee beans in a solvent to absorb the caffeine from the coffee in order to remove it. The solvent used is formaldehyde — which, by the way, is embalming fluid. I'll let that one sink in for a moment. And . . . because all decaf coffee still contains caffeine (just less of it), it still raises cortisol levels. Still think decaf is a good option? So here's the good news: within our Health Masters' family of trusted and beneficial products is a safe, all-natural alternative to caffeine and harmful stimulants . . . a product you can take without the possibility of becoming addicted as you would with caffeine, sleeping pills or tranquilizers . . . a product which acts like a protective shield against the damaging effects of stress.

A Product We Proudly Call **Health Masters' Adrenal Support** And that brings me back to a condition that may be behind that rundown feeling that millions of Americans struggle with daily. A condition with which you might even be struggling.   A condition called chronic fatigue syndrome (CFS). According to the Mayo Clinic, CFS has eight official symptoms, plus the central symptom that gives the condition its name:

- Fatigue
- Loss of memory or concentration
- Sore throat
- Enlarged lymph nodes in your neck or armpits
- Unexplained muscle pain that moves from one joint to another without swelling or red ness Headache of a new type, pattern or severity
- Unrefreshed sleep
- Extreme exhaustion lasting more than 24 hours after physical or mental exercise.

Compounding the CFS problem is a syndrome universally known as "adrenal burnout syndrome." Burnout refers specifically to a type of adrenal fatigue brought about by lifestyle factors such as working too hard or juggling too many activities.

Specifically, adrenal burnout syndrome is a low functioning or under activity of the adrenal glands. It may also be termed 'adrenal insufficiency' or 'adrenal exhaustion.' In most cases, the cause of 'burnout' is not a single shock to the system. Instead, it is usually a slow decline in adrenal activity due to nutritional deficiencies and the accumulation of toxic metals and chemicals in the body. As these causes are removed, the adrenal glands easily recover.

Adrenal burnout syndrome differs from simple fatigue in that burnout is not relieved by getting a few good nights' sleep, as is the case with fatigue. This is the case because adrenal exhaustion is not just a sleep deficit, although that may be an aspect of the syndrome. Burnout is a deeper derangement of the body's energy-producing system, of which fatigue is one symptom. Detecting Adrenal Burnout: Unfortunately, when a person complains to their doctor of fatigue, depression or other symptoms that are often related to the adrenal glands, most of the time the doctor neither asks the right questions nor runs tests of the adrenal glands. Instead, patients are told to take a vacation, are given an anti-depressant, or told it is "in their head." The right questions, however, would often be enough to assess the condition fairly accurately. These would include "How many hours of sleep are you getting". . . "Do you use caffeine or other stimulants" . . . and "What other symptoms are you having?" Let me explain how this can often identify adrenal burnout, even without other testing.

Signs and Symptoms:

A simple and quite reliable way to assess adrenal burnout in a general sense is with signs and symptoms. A common sign, for example, is a low blood pressure in the absence of other obvious causes.

Usually, a person will also often feel fatigued, even though he or she sleeps soundly. If you're not sleeping, the problem may simply be a sleep deficit. You may not feel tired, however, if you drink coffee, other caffeinated beverages or use other stimulants. Another common symptom is depression. Others include joint pain, cravings for sweets, pain in the lower back area and perhaps excessive thirst or craving for sweet and salty foods. Together these symptoms can help your doctor decide if you need further testing. From the moment you wake up till you finally go to sleep at night, your mind and body are bombarded with stressful stimuli. It could be a situation at work, the drive home or financial worries . . . pretty much any and everything. And when stress occurs, the body prepares to take action. This preparation is called the "fight-or-flight response." In the fight-or-flight response, levels of hormones — like cortisol — shoot up.

Cortisol is produced by the adrenal gland and increases blood sugar to ultimately make a lot of stored energy available to cells. These cells are then primed to help the body get away from danger. That's when the carb cravings hit and we find ourselves bingeing on sugary foods and drinks. Now your insulin levels are skyrocketing which leads to an increase in body fat, and ultimately, obesity and, in many cases, diabetes.

GET YOUR ADRENALS WORKING AGAIN:

If you're exhausted first thing in the morning or spend the day feeling tired . . . if you feel like you need to continue using caffeinated beverages and sugar to keep you going . . . if you're eating better than you have in years and managing to exercise a few days a week and still feel sluggish . . . it sounds like your body is trying to tell you something. And if you're genuinely concerned about the long-term impact from uncontrolled stress to your entire body (and you should be!), then it's time to take action.

So before you go to bed tonight only to find that you can't fall asleep and now you're worried that you'll wake up tired tomorrow — AGAIN — let's do something NOW to end this harmful cycle. It's time to re-energize your adrenal glands. It's Time For **Health Masters' Adrenal Support**.

Naturally Enhance Your Adrenal Cells:

For nearly a century doctors have relied on adrenal supplements to supercharge sluggish adrenal glands. But most of those supplements have been derived from synthetic sources and, as we're now discovering, are very unhealthy (especially glandular extracts which until I can find a pure source,

I will not recommend). The best source I have found for adrenal support is an aptogenic herbal remedy featuring extracts of cordyceps, rhodiola, and panax ginseng — all designed to support the stress response — as well as select B vitamins to support adrenal hormone production.

This is why **Health Masters' Adrenal Support** is formulated from 100% all-natural adrenal supporting concentrates. **Health Masters' Adrenal Support** is a unique formula containing concentrated mixtures of cordyceps, rhodiola, and panax ginseng to support adrenal production. These concentrates are carefully selected, processed to be free of hormones and chemicals, and combined in precise proportions to best facilitate building and maintaining healthy adrenal tissue and function. Most people notice a change in a few days, but for optimal effectiveness and to fully support and benefit your adrenal glands, you should continue taking Health Masters' Adrenal Support for at least six months.

My mother-in-law Shirley Bennett loves this product. Shirley is 78 years young and has the energy of a 40-year-old. Sharon and I also take this product daily. This stuff is amazing because it helps your body to naturally produce energy. You'll see. Just be sure to take it before noon. Taking this product before going to bed is not a good idea at all. It protects you from the physical dangers of stress.

What follows is a list and explanations of the physical damage stress can cause to all our different body parts:

The Brain: Beginning in the brain, stress causes a surge in hormones which results in intense alertness. In this state, we can neither sleep nor relax. Additionally, our mind cannot function at this extreme level for prolonged periods: Eventually the hormone surges and exhaustion causes tension headaches, irritability, aggression, inability to concentrate and memory loss. Unchecked stress can also trigger depression, which strikes twice as many women as men. Stress suppresses the hypothalamus, the emotion control center in our brains, curbing the production of the hormones that energize us and make us feel well. A lot of times a condition of "Brain Fog" can also develop. Health Masters' Adrenal Support contains a standardized extract of Cordyceps Sinensis which has been shown in several studies to possess anti-inflammatory, anti-tumor, anti-stress, antioxidant, mind-boosting, immune-enhancing, and rejuvenating properties. Many people report feeling energized with an overall sense of well-being.

The Ears: The surging hormones induced by stress improve our hearing to help us react to danger. But better hearing can actually be bad for the body: A Cornell University study concluded that even moderate noise elevates heart damaging stress hormones. Studies have also shown that a lot of small noisy stressors added together — honking horns, ringing telephones and loud co-workers — can be more dangerous to the body than one major stressful event.

The Lungs: One of the first things we do when we feel stressed is hyperventilate. It is part of the body's fight-or-flight response -- in case we are in danger and need the extra oxygen in our bloodstream to run for cover. Those quick breaths can cause dizziness and sharp pains in the diaphragm. Severe stress can aggravate asthma and other dangerous respiratory conditions.

The Eyes: The adrenaline rush from stress dilates the eyes, improving vision. But it also triggers eye ticks because eye muscles become fatigued. Eyes may bulge if stress over-stimulates the thyroid gland.

The Mouth: Dry mouth, bad breath and difficulty swallowing occur when stress makes us take short, shallow breaths. Under constant stress, some people clench their jaws or grind their teeth.

The Hair: The hair is considered a barometer of inner health, so hair is often the first to suffer. A body under stress burns nutrients like the vitamin selenium, and that can lead to dull hair and premature graying. Chronic stress can trigger the autoimmune system to attack hair follicles, causing hair to fall out completely or in clumps.

The Heart: A heart under stress pumps fast and hard. Blood pressure rises as the body produces the hormone epinephrine as well as the hormone cortisol. That can lead to heart palpitations and chest pains. In those with heart disease, stress can prevent blood from clotting properly and stimulate the formation of plaque that plugs arteries. Researchers say that even thinking about something stressful raises blood pressure. A Swedish study concluded that stressful romantic relationships were more damaging to a person's heart than work-related stress: Those in troubled marriages were three times more likely to be hospitalized for heart problems.

The Immune System: Did you ever get sick after a stressful event? Extreme and constant stress lowers our white blood cell count, making us more susceptible to disease and hampering our body's ability to heal itself. One study showed that the pneumonia vaccine was less effective in people under constant stress. Meanwhile, researchers are studying the link between stress and autoimmune disorders like Grave's disease, in which antibodies attack the thyroid, eye muscles and skin.

The Joints, Muscles and Bones: At tense moments, our brain sends messages to the muscles, tightening them and preparing them for action. Chronic stress can aggravate rheumatoid arthritis, cause sore muscles and make us prone to sprains. The Skin Stress causes hormones to be released that make acne, rashes and itchy patches worse. Some people blush, while others go pale when the small blood cells in the skin contract. Under extreme stress, people can become covered in hives. Any skin problem will get worse when you are under stress.

The Digestive System: Under stress, the brain shifts blood flow away from the digestive tract, which slows digestion. The result: indigestion, diarrhea, constipation, incontinence and colon spasm. Stress increases acid production, aggravating ulcers. It is also linked to colitis and irritable bowel syndrome, a painful and sometimes debilitating disorder, which is why it's critical after the age of 40 to also take **Health Masters' Digestive Enzyme**

Blend. Sharon and I both take one of these with every meal. It really does help with digestion problems, including acid reflux.

You can't avoid stress, but you surely can impact the way your body responds to it! Thousands of people suffer from stress and constant fatigue not relieved by rest and sleep. When this occurs, cortisol — the "stress hormone" — is released by the adrenal glands. Elevated cortisol related to CFS and adrenal burnout is not only linked to weight gain and sleep disorders, but it can seriously impair the immune system. Chronic infections may develop, thus setting the stage for colds, the flu and the development of several types of degenerative conditions.

Mental Stress And Anxiety Is Alleviated with **Health Masters' Adrenal Support** which also contains Rhodiola rosea root to combat the stress you encounter on a typical daily basis.

Rhodiola rosea is an essential component of all biological membranes and is required for normal cellular structure and function. The participation in physical activity often challenges a variety of physiological systems; consequently, the ability to maintain normal cellular function during activity can determine sporting performance. In addition to physical stress, Rhodiola rosea supplementation benefits those suffering from mental stress. Rhodiola rosea supplementation has been reported to improve the moods of healthy young adults when faced with a stressful mental task. Natural hormone production is increased.

B6 and Panothenic Acid are also key components of **Health Masters' Adrenal Support**.

These supplements support the adrenal gland, protecting it from stress, and help it maintain normal (not elevated or depressed) levels of cortisol in the body. This can be a helpful addition to the treatment of someone with chronic fatigue. **Health Masters' Adrenal Support** puts the missing 'oomph' back into your adrenal glands. In fact, its effect on you is not unlike putting fresh batteries in a fading lantern So now you can enjoy not just new energy, but also a renewed sense of well-being that you may have thought was long-gone, and levels of essential anti-Stress nutrients are maintained. When we're stressed, the need for nutrients is much greater. Carbohydrates, when excessive in the diet, stress the adrenals. Diets low in protein may also create deficiencies. Inadequate or poor quality water affects oxygenation of the tissues. Most diets are low in nutrients required by the adrenals. These include B-complex vitamins, vitamins A, C and E, manganese, zinc, chromium, selenium and other trace elements. The reasons for this begin with how food is grown. Most food is grown on depleted soils. Processing and refining further deplete nutrients.

Habits such as eating in the car or while on the run further diminish the value derived from food. Also, allergic reactions to foods such as wheat and dairy products can damage the intestines and reduce the absorption of nutrients. That's why **Health Masters' Adrenal Support** is packed with adrenal friendly B-vitamins to ensure that your healthy levels of these anti-stress nutrients are maintained.

STAY AWAY FROM HARMFUL ARTIFICIAL STIMULANTS!

If you've ever found yourself reaching for extra coffee, energy drinks, or herbal stimulants throughout the day, then you know the fake energy boost they provide doesn't last. Even worse: It's usually followed by an energy "crash" that leaves you feeling even more worn out than before. One secret to lasting energy I've learned is to start my morning with a good quality protein supplement. Which is why when I get up each morning, I begin my day with a glass of Health Masters' Fit Food Protein. It's an incredible stabilizer for blood sugar and has a low glycemic index. I love the stuff.

Stimulants put more than just the brain into overdrive. The effects on the body vary depending on several factors including your age, stress level, overall health, etc. But the biggest concern is the side effects of artificial stimulants. They can increase your heart rate and blood pressure, and in extreme cases, lead to heart attack or stroke.

Safely Reinvigorate Your Adrenal Glands! Try Health Masters' Adrenal Support Risk-Free So many people have told about the changes they've noticed with Health Masters' Adrenal Support, that I'm positive it can help you feel better, too. Youthful vigor . . . improved stamina . . . enhanced well-being. It can all be yours again. Here's how . . . "A Noticeable Surge In Your Energy Levels Or Your Money Back!" If you don't absolutely love what Health Masters' Adrenal Support does for you — especially at the start of your day or in the late afternoon when you typically crave sugary snacks — then just send back the unused portion of Health Masters' Adrenal Support and I'll refund your full purchase price.

Don't Let Uncontrolled Stress Control You! The medical community knows that stress is the biggest threat to your overall good health — and now you can do something about it withHealth Masters' Adrenal Support. As I stated earlier, you can't avoid stress, but you surely can impact the way your body responds to it. Give it a try today — you won't be sorry. I guarantee it!

I take it every morning after my Health Masters' Fit Food Protein. Just remember this . . . don't take it at night! As I've already mentioned, Health Masters' Adrenal Support naturally helps your body produce lots of energy — something you don't need before going to bed. Try Health Masters' Adrenal Support RISK-FREE with my 100% Money Back Guarantee: I guarantee that Health Masters' Adrenal Support will help you awaken and boost a sluggish energy to levels like you used to have! It sounds incredible because it truly is!

19 | Two Food Products That Can Destroy Brain and Lungs!

Brightly colored dried fruit, thick red juicy meats, and delicious wines perfectly preserved and calling out to you from your grocer's shelf, sometimes for months at a time. Colorful, beautiful and well-preserved poison . . . thanks to an unregulated, seriously harmful, potentially deadly, food additive.

SULFITES

For centuries, sulfites have been an accepted additive used to assist with the preservation of foods in various forms for centuries. And they have always been considered relatively safe by the United States Food and Drug Administration (FDA), so why I am talking about it now?

For two reasons: One, because they are considered a food additive rather than an ingredient, regulatory organizations such as the FDA, only require minimal labeling of foods that contain sulfites. According to the FDA, approximately one in 100 people is sensitive to sulfites in food, and the majority of these individuals are asthmatic, suggesting a link between asthma and sulfites. Individuals who are sulfite-sensitive are prone to experiencing headaches, breathing problems, and rashes — and in the most severe cases — cardiac arrest and death. That bag of dried tropical food isn't looking as appetizing now, is it? Unfortunately for the sulfite sensitive, dizzying arrays of foods contain added sulfites, in addition to those which may be naturally occurring. Wine and dried fruit are the two biggest culprits, but sulfites can also be found on vegetables and seafood. In most cases, a restaurant or grocery store will not know about the sulfite content of the food they sell, and, therefore, have difficulty assisting consumers with identifying potentially dangerous foods. In some cases, companies which target the sulfite sensitive have arisen, offering foods which are guaranteed to be sulfite free.

Wine is the food most people associate with sulfites, because it has longer stability and shelf life when sulfites are added. The fermentation process of wine also produces sulfites, so no wine can be truly sulfite-free. Organic wines must be produced without added sulfites, but for the sulfite sensitive, this does not eliminate the risk. Other foods such as dried fruit are sometimes sold in an "unsulfured" version, which means that they were produced without sulfites. Unsulfured dried fruit tends to be dull in color, and has a shorter shelf life, even though it is perfectly delicious.

Some things to watch for with sulfites:

Sulfites in food are not dangerous for most of the population, although they can lead to discomfort and allergies in varying amounts. Asthmatics should try to be careful with foods that may contain sulfites, and in all cases, if you visit a doctor because of an allergic reaction, make sure to detail what you have eaten in the last 24 hours. Most violent reactions to sulfites happen within an hour of consuming them, but it is better to err on the side of detail when it comes to allergies. The FDA estimates that one out of a hundred people is sulfite-sensitive, and that five percent of those who have asthma, are also at risk of suffering an adverse reaction to the substance. Complicating matters, scientists have not pinpointed the smallest concentration (response threshold level) of sulfites needed to provoke a reaction in a sensitive or allergic person. FDA requires food manufacturers and processors to disclose the presence of sulfite agents in concentrations of at least 10 parts per million, but the threshold may be even lower. The assay used to detect the level of sulfites in food is not sensitive enough to detect amounts less than 10 ppm in all foods (that's one part sulfite to 100,000 parts of food — the equivalent of a drop of water in a bathtub).

Watch for reactions to sulfites:

The most rapid reactions occur when sulfites are sprayed onto foods or are present in a beverage, but the most severe reactions occur when sulfites are constituents of the food itself, says one leading researcher. And while a person can develop sulfite sensitivity at any point in life, no one knows what triggers the onset or the mechanism by which reactions occur. Let me give you a personal example. Just recently my right arm started itching (Remember, I sent out an email telling people how to control or reduce dry itchy skin. I found that turmeric (**Turmeric Force**) and the GHI cleanse (**Health Masters' GHI Cleanse**) did a great job to stop the itching.) I started thinking that perhaps I had developed a food allergy. I went to see my family physician, Dr. Todd Robinson, and we did a simple blood test for allergies . . . and guess what? I had developed a tomato allergy. Since I stopped eating tomatoes, the itching has stopped. Eliminating tomato-based products was not a big deal for me as I never really cared for them or any other night shade vegetables: I've always been concerned with their inflammatory response in the body and how they contribute to rheumatoid arthritis.

Asthmatics beware:

Many doctors also believe that asthmatics could develop difficulty breathing by inhaling sulfite fumes from treated foods. In a severe reaction, an overwhelming degree of bronchial constriction occurs, causing breathing to stop. Once this occurs, oxygen is unable to reach the brain, heart, and other organs and tissues thus possibly producing a fatal heart rhythm irregularity. The most common forms of sulfite used by the food industry include:

- Sulfur dioxide
- Sodium sulfite
- Sodium and potassium metabisulfite
- Sodium, calcium or potassium bisulfite.

Uses for Sulfites Sulfur-based preservatives, or sulfites, have been used around the world for centuries. Below are some of the uses:

- Inhibit oxidation ("browning") of light-colored fruits and vegetables (dried apples and dehydrated potatoes)
- Prevent melanosis (black spots) on shrimp and lobster
- Discourage bacterial growth as wine ferments
- Condition dough
- Bleach food starches
- Maintain the stability and potency of some medications.

When the Federal Food, Drug, and Cosmetic Act were amended in 1958 to regulate preservatives and other food additives, the FDA considered sulfites to be Generally Recognized as Safe (GRAS). But when the FDA reevaluated their safety and proposed to affirm the GRAS status of sulfite agents in 1982, the agency received numerous reports from consumers and the medical community regarding adverse health reactions.

In 1985, the FASEB concluded that sulfites are safe for most people, but pose a hazard of unpredictable severity to asthmatics and others who are sensitive to these preservatives. Based on this report, the FDA took regulatory actions in 1986 and prohibited the use of sulfites to maintain color and crispness on fruits and vegetables meant to be eaten raw (for instance, restaurant salad bars or fresh produce in the supermarket). They also required companies to list on product labels sulfiting agents that occur at concentrations of 10 ppm or higher, and any sulfiting agents that had a technical or functional effect in the food (for instance, as a preservative) regardless of the amount present (This labeling requirement was extended to standardized foods such as pickles and bottled lemon juice in 1993.)

The FDA requires that the presence of sulfites be disclosed on labels of packaged food (although manufacturers need not specify the particular agent used). This information is included in the ingredient portion of the label, along with the function of the sulfiting agent in the food (for instance, a preservative).

When food is sold unpackaged in bulk form (as with a barrel of dried fruit or loose, raw shrimp (which you shouldn't be eating anyhow as it is on my top 10 List of Foods to Never Eat), store managers must post a sign or some other type of labeling that lists the food's ingredients on the container or at the counter so that consumers can determine whether the product was treated with a sulfiting agent.

In 1987, the FDA proposed to revoke the GRAS status of sulfiting agents on "fresh" (not canned, dehydrated or frozen) potatoes intended to be cooked and served unpackaged and unlabeled to consumers (French fries, for example), and issued a final ruling to this effect in 1990. However, the rule was held null and void in 1990 after a protracted court battle in which the "fresh" potato industry prevailed on procedural grounds.

SULFITES ALL AROUND US:

Since 1985, the FDA's Adverse Reaction Monitoring System has been tracking reactions to sulfites. Over a 10-year period, 1,097 such cases have been reported. Today, sulfites are still found in a variety of cooked and processed foods (including baked goods, condiments, dried and glazed fruit, jam, gravy, dehydrated or pre-cut or peeled "fresh" potatoes, molasses, shrimp, and soup mixes) and beverages (such as beer, wine, hard cider, fruit and vegetable juices, and tea). Since sulfites are added to so many foods, someone who is sensitive to the additive must not assume that a food is safe to eat. If the food is packaged, read the label. If it is being sold loose or by the portion, ask the store manager or waiter to check the ingredient list on the product's original bulk-size packaging.

Avoid processed foods that contain sulfites, such as dried fruits, canned vegetables, maraschino cherries, and guacamole. If you want to eat a potato, order a baked potato rather than hash browns, fries, or any dish that involves peeling the potato first. If you have asthma, have your inhaler with you when you go out to eat. Similarly, if you've experienced a severe reaction to sulfites in the past (such as breaking out in hives), carry an antihistamine and make sure you ask your doctor if he thinks it necessary for you to have a have handy a self-administering injectable epinephrine, such as EpiPen, so that if you have a reaction you can stabilize your condition until you get to an emergency room. Sulfites are also produced in our bodies as a byproduct of taurine, Cysteine and methionine — which all contain sulfur.

Sulfites are also generated by various white blood cells during infections to kill invading microorganisms (people with pneumonia have higher levels of blood sulfites which recede as the infection drops down.) Sulfite oxidase is an enzyme contained within our tissues which enables most people to be protected against bad reactions from sulfites. Typically, people have higher levels of this enzyme in their liver, kidneys, skeletal muscles, heart, and brain, and low levels in the thymus, spleen, leukocytes, colon, small intestine and lungs. Unfortunately, this enzyme decreases as a person ages or suffers from a chronic illness, making these people prone to severe toxic sulfite reactions. Babies born without this enzyme suffer from seizures, brain destruction, and abnormal brain development and, ultimately die.

The following examples of foods that may contain sulfites:

Baked goods, Soup mixes, Jams, Canned vegetables, Pickled foods, Gravies, Dried fruit, Potato chips, Trail mix, Beer and wine, Vegetable juices, Sparkling grape juice, Apple cider, Bottled lemon juice and lime juice, Tea, Many condiments, Molasses, Fresh or frozen shrimp, Guacamole, Maraschino cherries, Dehydrated, pre-cut or peeled potatoes.

Tackling headaches caused by sulfites:

Research points to a connection between migraine headaches and sulfites from foods — with wine, chocolate, and cheese as the main culprits . It is also well established that cheese — high in glutamate — is among the most aggressive triggers for migraines. (Note: studies show that during migraine attacks, spinal fluid glutamate (a measure of brain glutamate levels) rose significantly during the migraine attack and subsides once the attack has ended. There is another interesting link between migraine headaches, brain toxicity in general, and glutamate in the brain. It's been shown that the needed brain enzyme — glutamate dehydrogenase — is inhibited by high sulfite levels in the blood and tissues.

High brain glutamate leads to an adverse brain reaction called excitotoxicity, which can lead to headaches and possibly, Parkinson's, Alzheimer's and ALS, among others. As sulfite inhibits this crucial enzyme, more severe asthma attacks may be triggered. And because the majority of processed foods also contain high levels of glutamate additives, the combination of sulfites and glutamates make the toxic reaction more serious.

Is there a connection between brain damage . . . and sulfites?

Some researchers seem to think the list of havoc that higher levels of sulfites can wreak on the system of a person is pretty dreadful:

- Long-term damage to the nervous system
- On-going behavioral problems (depression, insomnia and anxiety, among others)
- Free radical production
- Chronic inflammation
- Neurodegeneration
- Cancer

Also, sulfites could make existing autoimmune and circulatory conditions even worse and cancerous conditions more deadly. The brain seems to be the most seriously affected by sulfites, as noted by recent research in rats. Rats start out with much higher sulfite oxidase than humans which is reduced to human levels. Studies revealed that sulfites:

- Reduced the gluthianone peroxidase in the brain (a symptom common among Parkinson's sufferers)
- Caused impaired function in the studied rats (including difficulty learning)
- Increased free radicals in the brain adversely which affected memory

Below are several clues that you may be sensitive to sulfites (which probably means your sulfite oxidase enzyme is down):

- You become tired after ingesting one of the foods, listed above, that contains sulfites
- One can look at the food label to see if the product contains sulfites
- You cough after ingesting sulfites, due to the impairment of the lung ATP energy
- You have asthma
- You develop low blood glucose (sugar) after ingesting sulfites (since sulfites disrupt the regulation of blood sugar)
- You get a headache after ingesting sulfites
- You experiences itching and reddening of the skin after ingesting sulfites contained in foods, drinks or drugs.

Also, sulfites can inhibit 90% of lung ATP energy production can impair liver cell ATP energy production, and can deplete glutathione (chemical that helps the liver filter the blood and helps protect cell enzymes from damage). Anything that reduces your production of ATP energy can cause fatigue.

Ways to Protect Yourself against Sulfite Toxicity: You're never going to be able to protect yourself against all sulfites but there are things you can do avoid — and perhaps even prevent the effects from becoming catastrophic. First, try to avoid drinking wine containing sulfites and cut back or eliminate the foods listed in this article. And remember, the severity of your reaction to sulfites will depend on the contributing factors which may already exist.

Factors affecting sulfite toxicity:

- The level of antioxidants you take in from your diet and supplements
- The level of your exposure to environmental toxins (where you live, work, etc.)
- How healthy you already are and any preexisting conditions
- The effectiveness of any detoxification system you current employ.

Differences in these factors also explain why some people are severely affected by sulfites, while others show no adverse reactions at all. There is evidence that Vitamin E (Health Masters' Super Potent E) blocks the toxic effects of sulfites, but not the brain impairment. Amino acid L-Leucine (Health Masters' GHI Cleanse) can activate glutamate dehydrogenase (and possibly lower brain glutamate.) · R-lipoic acid can reduce the brain toxicity of sulfites as it raises brain glutathione, an important antioxidant.

A list of the key vitamins and minerals needed to help protect the body against sulfite toxicity:

- High dose vitamin B12 (methylcobalamin) (Health Masters' Sublingual B12) - 5,000 mcg a day
- Thiamine HCL (vitamin B1) (Health Masters' GHI Cleanse) - 100 mg twice a day; sulfites destroy vitamin B1 in foods
- Riboflavin 5-PO4 (Health Masters' GHI Cleanse) - 50 mg twice a day
- Niacinamide (Health Masters' Insulin Support) - 500 mg twice a day
- Pyridoxal 5-PO4 (Health Masters' Corticare B5 B6) - 30 mg a day
- Folate (Health Masters' GHI Cleanse) - 400 mcg a day
- Natural Vitamin E (Unique-E) (Health Masters' Super Potent E) - 400 IU a day
- Tocotrienol (Health Masters' Super Potent E) - 50 mg twice a day
- Magnesium citrate/malate (Health Masters' Magnesium and Malate Acid) - 500 mg twice daily
- R-Lipoic acid - 50 mg twice daily with meals

The danger of your body's travelling amino acid:

It looks like the amino acid homocysteine is finally starting to gain traction within the traditional medical community. Doctors now recognize that very high levels of homocysteine put patients at an increased risk for coronary artery disease. Further, high homocysteine levels may make blood clot more easily than it should cause a clot inside your blood vessel — called a thrombus. A thrombus can travel in the bloodstream and get stuck in your lungs (called a pulmonary embolism), in your brain (which can cause a stroke) or in your heart (which can cause a heart attack.) The new thinking says that high homocysteine is a better indicator of heart attack than cholesterol levels. Keeping homocysteine levels low by using nutrients (B6 (**Health Masters' Corticare B5 B6**), B12 (**Health Masters' Sublingual B12**), folate (**Health Masters' GHI Cleanse**) and betaine (**Health Masters' GHI Cleanse**) and magnesium (**Health Masters' Magnesium and Malate Acid**), curcumin (**Health Masters' Dimension**), quertin (**Health Masters' HGH Stimulate**) and ellagic acid (**Health Masters' GHI Cleanse**)) can protect tissues. Homocysteine is normally changed into other amino acids for use by the body. If your homocysteine level is too high, you may not be getting enough B vitamins (**Health Masters' B Complex**) to help your body use the homocysteine. Most people who have a high homocysteine level don't get enough folate (also called folic acid), vitamin B6 (**Health Masters' Corticare B5 B6**) or vitamin B12 (**Health Masters' Sublingual B12**) in their diet. Replacing these vitamins often helps return the homocysteine level to normal. Other possible causes of a high homocysteine level include low levels of thyroid hormone, kidney disease, psoriasis, some medicines or when the condition runs in your family. Research points to homocysteine-producing metabolites in several tissues, producing free radicals, lipid peroxidation byproducts and powerful excitotoxins. One of the major metabolites — Cysteine acid — activates receptors resulting in excitotoxicity which ultimately leads to heart attacks, birth defects, heart failure and some cancers. Plastic Bottles Release Potentially Harmful Chemicals (Bisphenol A). After Contact with Hot Liquids When it comes to Bisphenol A (BPA) exposure from polycarbonate plastic bottles, it's not whether the container is new or old but the liquid's temperature that has the most impact on how much BPA is released, according to University of Cincinnati (UC) scientists. BPA is one of many man-made chemicals classified as endocrine disruptors, which alter the function of the endocrine system by mimicking the role of the body's natural hormones. Hormones are secreted through endocrine glands and serve different functions throughout the body. The chemical--which is widely used in products such as reusable water bottles, food can linings, water pipes and dental sealants — has been shown to affect reproduction and brain development in animal studies.

A team of researchers found when the same new and used polycarbonate drinking bottles were exposed to boiling hot water, BPA, an environmental estrogen, was released 55 times more rapidly than before exposure to hot water. Previous studies have shown that if you repeatedly scrub, dish-wash and boil polycarbonate baby bottles, they release BPA, telling us that BPA can migrate from various polycarbonate plastics. Bottles used for up to nine years released the same amount of BPA as new bottles. To conduct their tests, the researchers purchased commercially available polycarbonate water bottles. The bottles were subjected to seven days of testing designed to simulate normal usage during backpacking, mountaineering and other outdoor adventure activities.

It was discovered that the amount of BPA released from new and used polycarbonate drinking bottles was the same — both in quantity and speed of release — into cool or temperate water. However, drastically higher levels of BPA were released once the bottles were briefly exposed to boiling water. Because so many baby bottles are made of polycarbonate, one should be concerned over the release of toxins into baby's milk once the bottle is heated. Also of concern is that the women now bottle-feeding their babies use soy-based milk — another endocrine-disrupting concoction. Scientists continue to be baffled as to how these endocrine disruptors — including natural phyto-estrogens from soy which are often considered healthy — collectively impact human health, but a growing body of scientific evidence suggests it might be at the cost of one's health. Source: University of Cincinnati (2008, February 4) Organic Versus Industrial Foods. In the past few years shopping became much harder. Whether you're buying for a quick dinner for two or feeding the relatives on Sunday, now there's a decision to make: Do you buy healthy organic or cheap industrial?

If organic food weren't that expensive, the decision would be easy. Everybody would just consume organic food. But unfortunately, not everybody can afford it. Sometimes it looks like healthy food is becoming a luxury item. Or are some people just trying to earn big cash with organic food labels? The answer is a no-brainer. Just look at milk. One study said organically produced dairy products resulted in lower eczema in children. Organic apples? More antioxidant protection and less DNA damage than industrial apples. Industrial tomatoes? Lower levels of lycopene than organic tomatoes. Organic veggies? Packed with more powerful flavonoids than industrially produced foods . And the levels of harmful lipid peroxidation plummeted thanks to organic wines. I could go on, but I think you get the point: you can't beat the nutritional value of organically grown foods. You know the study I want to see? The one that covers the long- and short-term health effects of pesticides and herbicides left on fruits and veggies. That ought to be an eye opener.

And that should explain the increasing number of chronic diseases, cancers and developmental disorders in our country.

The Side Effects of Food Additives: Consider this: The transport of one form of glutamate (monosodium glutamate) is controlled by the Bioterrorism Act of 2002. Because there is so much concern about MSG, the FDA commissioned a study to be conducted by the Federation of American Societies for Experimental Biology (FASEB). The study resulted in a 350-page report completed on 31 July 1995 (which has since mysteriously been deleted from public archives).

The research determined that MSG consumption can result in the following side-effects:

- Burning sensation in the back of the neck, forearms and chest
- Numbness in the back of the neck, radiating to the arms and back
- Tingling, warmth and weakness in the face, temples, upper back, neck and arms
- Facial pressure or tightness
- Chest pain
- Headache
- Nausea
- Rapid heartbeat
- Bronchospasm (difficulty breathing) in MSG-intolerant people with asthma
- Drowsiness
- Weakness

Hidden Dangers in Your Food:

A majority of our best loved — and most successful food companies — use all kinds of chemicals and food additives to make our food look better, taste sweeter, last longer and line their pockets with huge profits. And who suffers? We do. Below is partial list of these so-called 'food grade' additives:

- High fructose corn syrup
- Omega-6 oils

Colorants Citrus Red 2 is carcinogenic and used to enhance the color of the skin in some Florida oranges and other fruits. Red dye #3; Studies were done in 1983 that showed thyroid tumors in rats on high amounts of this dye used in products that have a low moisture content such as tablets, or in high fat products, such as icing . FD&C Blue #1 — Brilliant Blue FCF was previously banned in many EU countries, but most have removed the ban. It is on the list of approved colorants in the U.S . FD&C Green #3 has been linked to studies showing tumors in rats that were injected with this dye. Tartrazine, also known as FD&C Yellow #5 or E-102; It provides the color yellow and as such, can also be found in green and blue candies. There is currently a petition to the FDA to ban tartrazine from food. This chemical has been linked to severe allergic reactions, especially in asthmatics and is one of the food additives thought to be a cause of hyperactivity in children. FD&C Yellow #6 — Sunset Yellow is Sudan 1 that has been sulfonated. Sudan 1 often remains as an impurity in Sunset Yellow. It may cause hyperactivity in children when combined with Sodium Benzoate. Ferrous Gluconate is a naturally derived, mineral colorant added to olives. It is also a medication used for treating anemia, and as a drug, has side effects, and contraindications. Preservatives Chlorphenesin and Phenoxyethanol: .The FDA has issued a consumer warning that these two substances cause depression of the central nervous system, vomiting and diarrhea in infants. Phenoxyethanol is used as a preservative in medications and cosmetics. BHA is a preservative used in cereals, potato chips and chewing gum to stop them from becoming rancid. The U.S. Department of Health and Human Services considers BHA to be a carcinogen and that it poses a reasonable risk to health.

Flavor Enhancers:

Aristolochic acid is an ingredient used in "traditional medicines" or "dietary supplements" that is known to potentially cause irreversible and fatal kidney failure. Sodium nitrate and nitrite are added to meats to stabilize them, give them their red color and provide that characteristic smoked flavor. Chloropropanols are a family of drugs commonly found in Asian food sauces like black bean, soy, and oyster sauce. Diacetyl, the chemical that imparts the buttery flavor in microwave popcorn has a disease named after it due to the large amount of microwave popcorn factory workers that came down with the lung condition... Diacetyl Induced Bronchiolitis Obliterans; or "Popcorn Worker's Lung." Potassium Bromate is a chemical added to flour to make bread rise better and give it a uniform consistency.

Some questions I have been asked:

Q: I've been taking omega-3 oils for two years. I recently became pregnant. Is omega-3 good for my baby?

A: Absolutely! Intake of dietary omega-3 fatty acids has been shown to have a number of important health benefits for developing babies and newborns — including giving them an edge in terms of early development. DHA (one of the two components of omega-3) (**Health Masters' Norwegian Omega 3**) is important for the developing brain, which accumulates large amounts of it during the first two years of life. Researchers found that infants born to mothers with higher blood levels of the omega-3 fatty acid docosahexaenoic acid (DHA) at delivery had advanced levels of attention spans well into their second year of life. Attention is an important component of intelligence early in life. In their first six months, these infant were two months ahead of those babies whose mothers had lower DHA levels. I recommend a daily dosage of 500 mg. for a pregnant woman. Adding a tablespoon daily of our cod liver oil (**Health Masters' Organic Blue Ice Cod Liver Oil**) in the third trimester has been shown to actually increase IQ scores.

Q: **I'm thinking of adding omega-3 to my regimen. I'm a 6' tall guy in relatively good health. How much should I be taking each day?**

A: Generally, I recommend at least 6 grams of omega-3 oils a day. (**Health Masters' Norwegian Omega 3**) I believe that omega 3 fatty acids are the one essential nutrient most missing in our modern day diet. This deficiency is now believed to play a major role in why so many people suffer from heart disease, cancers and brain disorders. The human body requires a tremendous amount of omega 3 fatty acids to function properly. In fact, the human brain is comprised of 60% fats, and approximately half of that fat is DHA omega 3.

Q: **Is it safe to take omega-3 with an anti-coagulant? If not, is there a supplement I should consider?**

A: You should never take omega-3 oils with an anti-coagulant without first consulting with your physician who gave you the drug. Ask him if you can try a natural approach using vitamin E (**Health Masters' Super Potent E**) and omega-3 oils. (**Health Masters' Norwegian Omega 3**) Here are a few supplements you can take in place of anti-coagulants from pharmaceutical companies (many of which have some very nasty side effects): Ginkgo biloba (**Health Masters' Memory Support**) acts on the blood vessels to improve blood flow, reduces platelet adhesion and neutralizes free radicals, all without side effects. Magnesium (**Health Masters' Magnesium and Malate Acid**) reduces abnormal blood clotting; People with high blood pressure usually have magnesium deficiency. Therefore, extra nutrients and mineral supplements with magnesium content are vital for them to avoid additional medical complications. Grape seed extract and pycnogenol also prevent abnormal blood clotting as it improves circulation, reduces inflammation, and controls blood sugar. It's also thought to strengthen blood vessels and improve visual function.

20 | Dead Doctors Do Not Lie: The Truth Revealed

Top Secrets Revealed How Doctors Sometimes Don't "Get It Right"

As the years pass and I find myself marking decades in the field of nutritional science, I am increasingly aware of two major facts—not opinions, FACTS:

1. There is a tremendous amount of Misinformation in circulation about what does, and does not contribute to health, or cause disease. Some people have believed errors for so long that it is almost impossible for them to face the truth. It is hard to get rid of old lies.

2. Much of this Misinformation is believed by people in the medical profession and in the media. Professionals in both of these areas tend to be highly reluctant to admit error or to adjust their beliefs, especially if they have held an opinion for a long time.

It's time to reexamine!

It's time to get current with the science!

It is time to confront the lies and half-truths.

Lies about Heart Disease and Strokes:

Former President Dwight Eisenhower, who served as President of the United States of America in the early 1950's, was a man well acquainted with heart problems. He had a number of heart attacks and eventually died of coronary heart disease. It is somewhat ironic, in retrospect, that at the time of his first heart attack, his cholesterol level was 164 mg/dl, which is considered "perfect" by today's standards. His weight was perfect, he exercised every day, and he had only occasional periods of mild hypertension.

The news about cholesterol theories was beginning to make headlines in the 1950's, and Eisenhower was quick to make sure that his cholesterol was measured—in fact, he had it measured ten times a year. He eliminated all saturated fats from his diet and ate what were considered heart-healthy dietary foods at that time, including margarine and corn oil. He reduced his intake of carbohydrates. And he did all these things at the recommendation of his cardiologists.

Eisenhower *should* have been in the lowest risk category for cardiovascular disease. He *should* have been very healthy. He died, nonetheless, from coronary disease.

The truth has been uncovered since Ike was in office. And the truth that we have known for *decades now*, is this:

There is no link between cholesterol levels, saturated fat, and heart disease.

Are you aware that the Japanese living in the United States have lower cholesterol levels than those living in Japan, yet they have higher heart attack rates than those living overseas? We find the same trend with Irish immigrants, African nomads, and the Navajo Indians—there is no linear relation between cholesterol levels and heart attack or stroke risk.

More than 50 years ago a well-known researcher at the time said that if Americans followed his recommended low-fat, high-carbohydrate diet—one high in polyunsaturated vegetable oils—heart disease and atherosclerosis would disappear by the year 2000. Diets improved—countless millions of people began to eat what was called a "heart healthy" diet, the year 2000 came and went, and heart disease and atherosclerosis are more widespread than ever.

During that time, statin cholesterol-lowering drugs were introduced, but at the end of the past two decades, the scientific evidence is clear: the overall rate of cardiovascular disease hasn't budged.

Looking back, it is very likely that the American Heart Association's recommendation that people switch from saturated fats to polyunsaturated vegetable oils may be responsible for more Americans being crippled or killed than in both World Wars combined. Sadly, these oils were also recommended by government health agencies and the media. The truth is that these oils increase the growth and spread of a number of cancers and are considered by many to be cancer's "fertilizers." In the nutritional research community, we have known this truth about polyunsaturated oils since the 1970s. Newer studies are linking these polyunsaturated vegetable oils—and others called partially hydrogenated oils—to many other diseases, including Alzheimer's disease and various neurodegenerative diseases. Not only do these oils cause tremendous cardiovascular damage, but also brain damage!

The famous Framingham Heart Study, reported internationally in the British medical journal called *The Lancet*, noted that men with cholesterol below 190 mg/dl **tripled** their risk of developing colon cancer when compared to those with levels greater than 200 mg/dl. Even lower rates of death following a first heart attack were found to be unrelated to cholesterol levels. There was no difference in the rates between men with levels a 180 mg/dl or lower, and those with levels greater than 250 mg/dl.

For the most part, reductions in heart attack rates and deaths were very small when it came to cholesterol's influence. One study, called the Multiple Risk Factor Intervention Trial (MRFIT) found only a .4 percent reduction in risk for those who followed a strict, low-cholesterol diet. Less than half of one percent is barely significant!

A Harvard study found that people with multiple risk factors for cardiovascular disease might gain three days to three months additional life if they avoided saturated fats. A University of California/San Francisco study found an increased life expectancy of three to four months. A McGill university study found that a low saturated-fat diet would increase life expectancy from four days to two months. These lengths of time are certainly not what the cholesterol-reducing authorities predicted forty or fifty years ago!

A great deal of misleading and misinterpreted data surrounded the hyped -up claims about cholesterol. For example, one drug company stated in bold type that its statin drug lowered heart attack risk by 36 percent. But check the fine print! There, the risk falls just one percent!

Taking vitamins C and E (**Health Master's Excellent C and Super Potent E**) reduce risk by a much greater percentage! When these and other supplements are combined with a proper diet and exercise, the risk dramatically drops, no drugs needed. Of course, this information is devastating to those who sell drugs, and you can be assured, they will do their utmost to protect their profit margins, even if it means the nation's overall health is reduced. In fact, when the prestigious medical journal JAMA (*Journal of the American Medical Association*) planned to report this news about nutritional approaches to lowering heart attack risk, the government tried to stop the publication of the studies (no doubt because pharmaceutical company lobbyists had protested). To its credit, JAMA refused and the scientific study was published.

Many people, including many physicians, believe that the discovery of various subtypes of fats — such as LDL-cholesterol — is a fairly recent finding. In fact, LDL-cholesterol was discovered in 1950 by Dr. John Gofman, a professor of medical physics at the University of California. Gofman found that it was the triglyceride level, not cholesterol level that was most closely linked to heart disease and atherosclerosis. By 1960, other confirming studies had been published to support his findings. These studies, however, were largely squelched. Why, because triglycerides are related to SUGAR and refined carbohydrate intake, not cholesterol or fat.

To report these findings widely would have been an admission that the high-carbohydrate diet widely advocated was an error!

Of course, the triglyceride findings explain why diabetics, who often have normal or low levels of cholesterol, still have a high incidence of heart disease and stroke. Unfortunately, the American Diabetes Association continues to recommend a high carbohydrate diet for diabetics—just as it has recommended for decades.

Let me repeat what we know to be TRUE: A diet that is low in saturated fats, and high in sugars and refined carbohydrates lowers HDL cholesterol and raises triglycerides and VLDL cholesterol—and this is the very pattern most associated with cardiovascular and stroke risk, especially among older people. We need to be encouraging people to lower their sugar and refined carbohydrate intake!

Although it doesn't seem to make sense to those untrained in blood chemistry and physiology of fats, a high HDL is much more important for your protection than the high total cholesterol is a risk.

21 | The Dangers of High Sugar and High Processed Diet

Studies have shown us that there are two subtypes of LDL-cholesterol. One is a "small dense" LDL, and the other is a large "buoyant" LDL. Actually, these sub-types of LDL were discovered more than forty years ago, although there seem to be many physicians who think this is a fairly new finding.

The small dense LDL particles, which are actually made of a protein called Apo B, are the most potentially harmful. And what produces this type of LDL? Sugars and refined carbohydrates! Saturated fats are known to increase LDL levels slightly, but saturated fats impact the protective larger buoyant LDL particles! Sugars and refined carbohydrates increase triglycerides, and increase the concentration of Apo B.

There is a simple test to determine the amount of Apo B in a person's bloodstream, and this test presents much better risk information than a total LDL-cholesterol test.

SUGAR AND METABOLIC SYNDROME

Years ago, the medical community believed that there were two types of diabetes—insulin dependent and insulin independent. In both types, insulin was thought to be deficient. Then in 1965 noted scientists Rosalyn Yalow and Solomon Aaron Berson discovered that some diabetics actually had too much insulin. They concluded that insulin resistance was the problem, and that it was due to faulty receptors within the tissues. The idea was slow to catch on. Two decades later, we know much more about this, and we also know that the greatest increase in the incidence of diabetes is among those with insulin resistance. This is now called Type 2 diabetes.

Not everybody who has insulin resistance has been diagnosed as diabetic—a large number of people have this resistance, but it remains undetected. The danger is that insulin resistance—also called Hyperinsulinism—is closely connected to atherosclerosis (hardening of the arteries). The process is this: Insulin promotes inflammation within many tissues, including blood vessels. The central process in atherosclerosis is chronic inflammation of the blood vessels.

Studies in animals have confirmed that animals fed a high-cholesterol diet, but with low insulin levels, had little atherosclerosis. When insulin was added to the high-cholesterol diet, atherosclerosis developed...substantially. The difference was the insulin, not the cholesterol!

All of this is related to a disorder that came to be called Syndrome X. It was first identified in 1987, but its relationship to cardiovascular disease risk wasn't substantiated until later. Now, Syndrome X is called Metabolic Syndrome. Researchers estimate that more than 45 million Americans have this disorder. It is growing in children at a rapid rate. The three main things associated with Metabolic Syndrome are:

1. **A diet high in sugar and refined carbohydrates.** As far back as 1931, researchers named John Peters and Evelyn Man measured cholesterol levels in 79 diabetic patients and found that only 9 of them had elevated cholesterol levels. They followed these subjects, and in 1962, found that their subjects had a 40 percent increase in triglyceride levels and a dramatic increase in the number of diabetics with atherosclerosis. Overall medical statistics confirm that in the 1930s only 10 percent of diabetics had atherosclerosis, but in the late 1950s, 56 percent had atherosclerosis-related diseases.
2. **A magnesium deficiency. (Health Master's Magnesium Glycinate)**
3. **Being exposed to MSG and other food excitotoxin additives early in life.** Lab animals that have been given too much MSG shortly after birth display the same changes in blood lipids that are seen in humans with Metabolic Syndrome: insulin resistance, high triglyceride levels, high VLDL levels, and hypertension. One study using rats found that exposure to just a few doses of MSG early in life increased free-radical generation within the walls of arteries for months (equivalent to decades in humans). MSG also lowered the level of protective antioxidant enzymes in arteries, something seen in people with coronary heart disease.

Recent studies have shown that insulin resistance is closely linked to a number of diseases, including cancer, Alzheimer's disease, and other degenerative disorders. Other studies have shown a strong correlation between high sugar intake and these same diseases. A high intake of sugar and refined carbohydrates alters the metabolism of a number of lipids (fats), which leads to heart disease, atherosclerosis, and diabetes. Too much insulin turns out to be very harmful!

Apart from changes in diet, one of the things most beneficial to reducing insulin is exercise. Actively working muscles use blood sugar (glucose) without insulin, and this helps lower both blood sugar and insulin levels in the blood. (**Health Master's Insulin Support**)

The Identifying Characteristics of Metabolic Syndrome:

Metabolic Syndrome is diagnosed if a person has a group of risk factors that include:

- Abdominal obesity, excessive fat tissue in and around the abdomen (sometimes called "beer gut")
- Elevated blood pressure
- Insulin resistance or glucose intolerance—which means the body cannot properly use insulin or blood sugar
- Atherogenic dyslipidemia or blood-fat disorders—high triglycerides, low HDL cholesterol and high LDL cholesterol—that foster plaque buildup in artery walls
- A pro-inflammatory state, such as elevated C-reactive protein in the blood

NOT ALL SUGARS ARE ALIKE

There are two types of sugar that have seen massive consumption in the last hundred years: sucrose and high-fructose corn syrup (called HFCS-55).

Sucrose is a refined product that has glucose and fructose. HFCS-55 has 55 percent fructose and 45 percent glucose. Fructose is highly reactive in the body—and unfortunately, it is often recommended to diabetics as a "safe sugar!"

In the body, excess sugar interacts with proteins and amino acids in a chemical process called glycation. Over time, these chemicals form even more complex chemicals called "advanced glycation end products"—also known as AGEs. Diabetics, especially, seem to form large amounts of these destructive products, which can be measured by a test called hemoglobin A1c.

People with Alzheimer's disease and Parkinson's disease have high levels of AGEs in the affected parts of their brains. AGE's generate huge amounts of free radicals and lipid peroxidation products that damage cells and tissues. Extensive free-radical damage is linked, in the end, to heart disease, strokes, diabetes, hypertension, and neurodegenerative diseases (such as Parkinson's and Alzheimer's). Some researchers are theorizing that it is the AGE's that cause diabetics to age so rapidly.

AGE's and free radicals both trigger intense inflammatory reactions, and this involves the immune system. Scientists who measure inflammation have found that high levels of inflammatory markers (called by such names as TNF-alpha, IL-6, CRP, and IL-1) predict more accurately who is at a greater risk of a stroke or heart attack than cholesterol levels. Inflammation studies are also better predictors of who is at the greatest risk of a heart attack after a coronary bypass or stent operation.

A diet high in sugar and refined carbohydrates dramatically increase the growth of belly fat—also called visceral fat. This fat in the abdomen secretes large amounts of inflammatory chemicals.

The Inflammation Factor:

Inflammation has been linked to gum disease, heavy metals (such as mercury, lead, and cadmium), chronic infections, Alzheimer's disease, and cardiovascular disease. It is the inflammation that oxidizes cholesterol and other fats leading to the arterial "crud" that is associated with atherosclerosis.

Oxidized LDL-cholesterol and other oxidized fats also damage brain cells.

Although oxidized LDL-cholesterol gets most of the blame, it is actually the oxidized lipids that are at the root of most of this arterial "crud." Omega-6 or N-6 oils (corn, safflower, sunflower, peanut, canola, and soybean oils) are the oils the government health agencies and American Heart Association have recommended for years. In fact, these are the very oils that are oxidized most quickly in the arteries, creating a chronic inflammation problem that can lead to the eruption of plaques and creation of blood clots that kill.

Visceral or abdominal fat has been shown to release increased amounts of inflammatory cytokines, which worsen inflammation.

At present, nearly 100 Americans are insulin resistant and nearly 20 million are full diabetic. These people are the ones at greatest risk of cardiovascular disease. And there is little question that excessive sugar and refined carbohydrate consumption is the major underlying problem—not a diet high in saturated fats or cholesterol.

22 | What Can Be Done About AGE?

As stated earlier, AGE's—also called the browning or Maillard reaction—occurs when foods high in sugar content are consumed in excess. Such foods include potatoes—with French fries and potato chips two of the major culprits.

The supplements that help reduce AGE formation are curcumin and quercetin, as well as these plant extracts: ellagic acid, berberine, silymarin, hesperidin, and green and white tea extract. (**Health Master's GHI Cleanse**) These all help reduce AGEs and improve blood sugar metabolism. Alpha-lipoic acid (**Health Master's Alpha Lipoic Acid**) a powerful antioxidant and hypoglycemic substance—also improves insulin resistance and helps with diabetes.

A recent study found that a lipid soluble form of vitamin B-1 (thiamine), (**Health Master's B Complex**) called benfotiamine is very efficient in clearing AGEs from the body. In this study, researchers fed a meal of chicken, potatoes, and carrots cooked in vegetable oil to 13 adults with Type 2 diabetes. They measured blood vessel function and they found that AGEs profoundly interfered with the function of both large arteries and microscopic blood vessels. The subjects in the study who were given benfotiamine were completely protected from the AGEs.

Benfotiamine (**Health Master's B Complex**) has been shown to reduce insulin resistance and act as an antioxidant. AGEs activate the release of C-reactive protein and thus, promote inflammation. The common form of vitamin B-2 does not have this effect.

Yet another way to cut down on AGEs, as well as oxidized fats, is to avoid using all polyunsaturated vegetable oils. Instead, use extra virgin olive oil or extra virgin coconut oil. To add another layer of protection, sprinkle one or more of these antioxidant spies in the oil and on foods: turmeric, cumin, and ginger.

Key tests that reveal potential problems:

Many people have been given so-called "cholesterol" blood tests. The better gauge is a test that takes a look at triglycerides, LDLSD and Apo B. This is called the Atherogenic triad in medical circles. In addition, you need to have a C-reactive protein test done to measure your level of inflammation. Other helpful tests are ones that check homocysteine levels, fibrinogen levels, and lipoprotein (a) levels. These tests identify independent risk factors that have more to do with heart attack and stroke risk than cholesterol levels.

Of course this is just a start. Call my office for more detailed supplement guidelines.

Supplements:

- Health Master's Ultimate Multiple
- Health Master's B Complex
- Health Master's Alpha Lipoic Acid
- Health Master's Insulin Support
- Health Master's Magnesium Glycinate
- Health Master's Super Potent E
- Health Master's Excellent C

All of these high quality supplements can also be purchased by calling my office at 1-800-726-1834.

°This information has not been evaluated by the Food and Drug Administration. Neither the information, nor any formula(s) mentioned are intended to diagnose, treat, cure or prevent any disease.

23 | Hair Loss in Men and Women, Plus Natural Way to Get Rid of Gray Hair

Zinc is critically important for men. There are several reason zinc is so important. I will briefly cover a few of the reasons.

Zinc is a key player in health. Overall it is at the top of that list for immune function. Along with boosting the production of immune system cells that attack infection-causing organisms, zinc enhances the ability of those cells to keep on fighting. Zinc also increases the body's supply of infection-fighting T-cells.

Zinc is in demand; in fact, it is necessary for the activity of about 100 enzymes in the body and is required for cell division. The production of proteins and DNA also depend on zinc, and wounds heal better when there's enough zinc in the body. You can also thank zinc if you have a normal sense of smell and taste.[1]

ZINC FOR MEN

Now let's explore why zinc is such a critical nutrient for men:

Supports testosterone levels.

Experts have known that a significant zinc deficiency is associated with abnormally low testosterone levels, but what about mild to moderately low zinc? A research team at Wayne State University School of Medicine evaluated 40 men (ages 20 to 80) and their zinc and testosterone levels. The authors induced marginally low zinc in young men and provided zinc supplements to elderly men who were zinc-deficient. They discovered that limiting zinc intake for 20 weeks caused a decline in testosterone levels and

that zinc supplements given for six months improved testosterone production.
[2]

Back in 1981 when I first started my company I quickly became known as the go to guy when men had problems with ED. **Remember I didn't have HGH stimulate back then so it was necessary to develop a protocol for ED that worked. I found that 50 mgs of zinc combined with 1600 IU of natural vitamin E corrected the ED in most cases.** The craziest thing I learned back in the 80's was that many men were dealing with ED in their 20s and 30s. Today ED is much WORSE!

Promotes healthy sperm:

Healthy, active sperm is essential for men who want to be fathers, and zinc plays a critical role in not only promoting sperm production but in regulating the motility (ability of sperm to swim) as well. A study in the *Proceedings of the National Academy of Sciences of the United States of America* reported on the importance of zinc in ensuring healthy sperm, noting that zinc "is an essential trace element for the maintenance of germ cells [immature sperm cells], the progression of spermatogenesis [sperm formation], and the regulation of sperm motility."[3]

Back in the 90's my wife was having difficulty getting pregnant. Her mother had taken DES when pregnant with Sharon.

One of the protocols we had to do was to have my sperm count checked. When the Doctor came in with the results he was amazed. He said "you have the most potent sperm sample I have ever seen". I explained to him it was the zinc and vitamin E I was taking. He didn't pay any attention to the facts I had given him. So I will say this one more time. Men, if you have poor quality sperm and your wife can't get pregnant or if you have a low or non existent sex drive take **Super Potent E and Zinc**. Viagra can cause blindness and deafness.

Protects the prostate:

Guess which nutrient is found in high concentrations in the prostate? Although zinc is present throughout the body, the prostate is second only to bone for high levels of zinc in males. Scientists are still exploring the significance of zinc in the prostate, but thus far they've found that men with low dietary zinc tend to be at greater risk for an enlarged prostate (benign prostatic hyperplasia, BPH) and prostatitis (inflammation of the prostate), and possibly prostate cancer. For example, a 2007 study reported that men who had prostatitis or prostate cancer had lower concentrations of zinc than healthy men. An Oregon State University study found that zinc could be an important factor in "regulating cell growth and apoptosis [cell death] in hyperplasia cells. I have also found over the years that men who take zinc on a regular basis do not seem to have problems in this area.

Helps prevent hair loss:

Zinc deficiency is seen in a significant number of people who suffer with alopecia, which can range from minimal hair thinning to complete baldness. Could taking zinc supplements help? A study of 15 individuals (10 men) with alopecia looked at this question. All the participants were given 50 mg per day of zinc for 12 weeks, and by the end of the study, nine participants had experienced hair growth. Zinc levels had increased more in the subjects who had hair growth than in those who did not respond to treatment. In addition to this benefit zinc, when combined with active B vitamins, seems to reduce gray hair.

You can also try our **Bao-Shi natural hair growth** for addition hair support.

How much Zinc?

The recommended daily allowance of zinc for men is 11 mg (it is 8 mg for women). I personally believe that this is way too low. Zinc is too important to be deficient. I have been taking 50mgs a day for over 30 years. My wife takes 30mgs a day.

Sources

[1]Dietary Supplement Fact Sheet: Zinc
    http://ods.od.nih.gov/factsheets/Zinc-HealthProfessional/
[2]Zinc status and serum testosterone levels of healthy adults.
    http://www.ncbi.nlm.nih.gov/pubmed/8875519
[3]Zinc is an essential trace element for spermatogenesis.
    http://www.ncbi.nlm.nih.gov/pmc/articles/PMC2705534/
[4]Zinc levels in prostatic fluid of patients with prostate pathologies.
    http://www.ncbi.nlm.nih.gov/pubmed?term=zinc%20and%20benign%20prostatic%20
    AND%20Gomez
[5]Differential response to zinc-induced apoptosis in benign prostate hyperplasia and prostate
    cancer cells.
    http://www.ncbi.nlm.nih.gov/pubmed/19576751
[6]The therapeutic effect and the changed serum zinc level after zinc supplementation in alopecia
    areata patients who had a low serum zinc level.
    http://www.ncbi.nlm.nih.gov/pmc/articles/PMC2861201/T

24 | Red Bull™ Alternative: No caffeine, Massive Energy Drink!

The Circulation-Boosting Secret of the 2012 Olympic Athletes

Read on to discover how to turn a plain glass of distilled water into a Superfood Cocktail that can help…

- Blood Pressure and Blood Flow…
- Alertness, Energy and Mood…
- Stamina and Performance…
- Mental Fatigue, Brain Function and Focus…

Something strange happened at the 2012 Olympics in London…

Athletes were spotted drinking a deep red "elixir" that they claimed would give them a natural (and legal) performance boost — and a competitive edge in winning the games.

A blog post by Canadian cross-country skier Sheila Kealey revealed that almost all of Team Canada's marathoners — including Dylan Wykes — were drinking it.

So was British marathoner Mo Farah and the entire U.K. Olympic team. And even U.S. competitors were caught drinking it as well.

But did this mysterious red "nectar" really boost their athletic performance? I'll let you be the judge…

Canada's Dylan Wykes made a top-20 finish in the men's Olympic marathon — the best finish for his country.

Mo Farah won a gold medal for the U.K. in the men's 10K race.

And the U.K. team won more Olympic medals than they have any time in history.

They all give the credit for their amazing wins to the sweet, red juice they drank while training and competing.

Now the big question is…

What performance-enhancing drink can turn Olympic athletes into Olympic Champions?

The answer is simple…

…**Beet juice!** Remember several months ago I was promoting the use of organic non GMO whole beets for consumption.

Well, many of you have contacted me and asked me when Healthmasters. com would start carrying the whole beets.

My search for the best beets on the planet have led me to a superfood of superfoods. Organic, non- GMO Crystallized beet juice.

So Yes, the juice from beets was all the rage with the 2012 Olympic athletes.

And Yes it is as incredible as eating whole beets… probably even better.

In fact many of the Olympic athletes have credited it with giving them the stamina and performance boost they needed to edge out their competitors — and win.

So perhaps you're not an Olympic athlete and wondering "Why should you care about beet juice?"

It's simple, if beet juice is such a boom to athletes and their performance… just imagine what it can do for your own circulation and energy levels!

As you know, I'm a university trained biochemist and have written extensively on nitric oxide. I am also a former college professor, lecturer, speaker educator, and international best- selling author .

The problem is with me promoting this new product as good as it is…

If you're like most people, you don't like the taste of beets. I personally love them but not liking them is totally understandable, but I need you to hang in there with me for a few minutes.

Because I'm going to reveal to you how you can experience all the tremendous benefits of beets — without that beet taste.

HEALTHMASTERS ORGANIC NON GMO BEET CRYSTALS:

Boosts Circulation Promising Healthy Blood Pressure and Increased Energy and Stamina!

If you're concerned about circulation, blood pressure, digestion, mental fatigue, a lack of stamina—or any of the many signs of aging… it is possible adding beet juice to your healthy diet can make a real, meaningful difference in your health.

And it might just surprise you to hear that beets are packed with more performance enhancing nutrients than any other vegetable at the dinner table—making beets perhaps the most effective super-food of the 21st century...

And, currently the hottest topic in health journalism...

Blood Pressure: According to a recent study published by *Nutrition Journal* drinking an 8 oz glass of beet juice helped lower blood pressure over 24 hours of drinking it. Researchers noted that further research is indicated to determine whether it would have a same effect over time if taken on a daily basis.

Brain Function: The *Journal Natural News* reported that scientists discovered drinking beet juice can increase blood flow to the brain helping with mental fatigue, focus and alertness.

Stamina: Published in the *Journal of Applied Physiology*, The University of Exeter found that beet juice increases exercise capacity in trained athletes by 16% when consumed before exercise. Some experts believe this may mean greater physical performance with less fatigue.

And clinical evidence is mounting to support the humble beets health boosting claims...

...that's because beet juice is a rich, natural source of dietary nitrate.

In fact, researchers have discovered that beets contain one of the richest food sources of nitrate.

And this is NOT the food additive known as "sodium nitrite"—you've been told is bad-for-you—used to preserve deli meat, hot dogs and bacon.

This nitrate is naturally found in beets and other plant sources. It converts in your body to nitric oxide.

Nitric oxide (N-O) has been making the headlines lately for its role in supporting healthy blood pressure and promoting a healthy cardiovascular system.

Researchers have found that it helps blood vessels to relax and widen... which can improve blood flow... allowing more oxygen rich blood to reach your heart... lungs... brain... sexual organs... and muscles.

Discover Nitric Oxide...IT

- **Was Awarded the Nobel Prize** in Physiology of Medicine for its discovery...
- **Helps The Body Dilate Blood Vessels** and veins, improving circulation...
- **Improves Oxygen Delivery** allowing for increased athletic endurance...
- **Helps The Body Improve Muscle Blood Flow** for better delivery of fuel...

- **Means That Athletes Can Accomplish More Work With Less Oxygen** and calories burned…
- **Is Considered By Some Scientists To Be As Important As Oxygen** to the human body.

"The discovery of nitric oxide and its function is one of the most important in the history of cardiovascular medicine."
— Dr. Valentin Fuster, Past President of the American Heart Association (as quoted in the *New York Times*).

WHY BEETS?

Our Superior Beets BEAT the Competition!

As far back as ancient Rome and Greece, beets have been faithfully cultivated for their outstanding ability to support health, performance and longevity. But recently, beets have been newsworthy because they are found to be a rich source of dietary nitrate. The body reduces nitrate for the generation of nitric oxide (N-O). N-O is responsible for the dilation of blood vessels, thus increasing blood circulation and oxygen delivery to cells. This results in improved maximum oxygen uptake (VO2Max) and oxygen efficiency, which determine an athlete's capacity for sustained exercise and endurance.

This is why its so important to take before a workout. Its gives me an incredible pump and longer endurance. My wife and son also love this product and use it in their pre-workout.

Healthmasters organic beet crystals are a superior and natural source of dietary nitrate that helps the body significantly increase physical endurance. It's delicious… and more nutritious and efficient than drinking large bottles of beet juice.

The Nobel Prize Winning "Miracle Molecule"

As I explained the human body uses nitrates for the generation of nitric oxide (N-O). N-O is the "miracle molecule" responsible for helping to support your arterial health and circulation while helping to keep your cells oxygenated.

The benefits of maintaining healthy N-O levels are endless…

- Healthy blood pressure…
- Enhanced stamina…
- Improved libido and enjoyment…
- Higher energy levels…
- Sounder sleep…

- Better focus and concentration…
- And so much more
- My wife Sharon told me to tell you since starting this product she has had a massive energy surge. Funny thing is she already had great energy.

Three researchers received the prestigious Nobel Prize for this ground-breaking discovery. Louis J. Ignarro, one of the prize winners says, "There may be no disease process where this "miracle molecule does not have a protective role."

The American Heart Association published one of many studies showing that Americans over 40 don't produce enough N-O. In fact, your body produces less than half of what you did when you were 20. And poor sleep — that frequently occurs as you age — further depletes the body's N-O levels.

Healthmasters Organic Beet crystals provide Three Times the N-O Power Without the Taste of Beets!

To get the astounding results of the folks in the studies, you'd have to drink a half liter of beet juice — that's 16.9 ounces — a day.

Or you'd have to go through the mess and hassle of juicing a bushel of beets yourself.

I did by the way find a great source for whole organic beets. If you still want them I can get them for you, but this is a lot easier and a lot less money and hassle.

Would you like to realize these same benefits… healthy blood pressure, circulation, increased libido, and mental function? *Absolutely!*.

But you draw the line at beets. You just can't get past that beet taste.

Well, I've got a question for you…

What if you can get the beet goodness without the beet taste… would you give it a shot?

To me this product tastes more like raspberries than beets.

INTRODUCING HEALTHMASTERS' BEET CRYSTAL CONCENTRATE.

…We've created the BEST beet product you're going to find anywhere.

These concentrated beet crystals help increase N-O levels without the need to drink 500ml of beet juice.

Healthmasters beet concentrate has been formulated to help your body deliver the highest level of N-O potential, so you can support healthy circulation, brain function and blood pressure.

What is its secret?

1) Highest quality, organic non GMO beets:

These are the ONLY beets we use in Healthmasters Beet Concentrate crystals assuring the highest quality... nutrients... and N-O generating power. No other beet juice on the market can make that claim!

2) Patented drying process:

Most companies use high heat to process beats — and that can destroy much of the nutrient content. Not ours. Our organic beet crystals are dried with an exclusive, patented low-heat drying process that preserves the beets' nutrients and nitrates .

As I mentioned above, the beets we use are richer in nitrates than other beets to start with. Thanks to this patented drying process, we are able to preserve those levels.

And Healthmasters Beet Concentrate contains the N-O boosting equivalent of 3 Organic Beets or 3 glasses of commercial Beet Juice all in an easy to mix rich-colored, concentrated crystal powder.

I've really just scraped the surface on the amazing health benefits of beets in this special report. But beets do so much more for your health that I want to tell you about... so you can truly tap into their healing power.

Healthier Circulation... Blood Flow... Blood Pressure... Brain Function... And Stamina! Not to Mention More Energy... Increased libido... And Endurance!

I'm sure you can tell how excited we are about beets... and in particular our great tasting, easy-to-use concentrated organic beet crystal formula... and it's super N-O boosting potential to support your healthy circulation, blood pressure, brain function and so much more.

BEETS FIGHT DISEASE AND PROMOTE HEALTH:

Beets can rejuvenate nearly every system of the body. Hardly any other vegetable can compare to the natural benefits of beets. Here are just a few of the many known capacities of beets:

- Accelerating bile secretion
- Accelerating cell replacement and restoring cell nucleus
- Boosting mood
- Boosting strength and stamina
- Lowering body temperature

- Preventing cold and flu
- Promoting healthy nails, shiny hair and smoother skin
- Purifying and detoxifying the liver, kidneys, and bladder
- Strengthening blood
- Regulating blood pressure
- Relieving constipation
- Removing toxins from the brain
- Speeding the formation of red corpuscles (and thus improving cellular oxygenation)
- Stimulating the immune system
- Strengthening skin and vein walls
- Improving the immune system

Ultimately, the effectiveness of beets is best used as a preventative disease protocol, when its highest value can halt the progression of a disease. If you're ready to boost your overall health with beets, then you are in good company.

Longstanding have ancient Romans enjoyed beet juice to daily maximize their health. Beet therapy treats specific health problems in a multitude of ways. **Today, even Dr. Mehmet Oz, and other natural health experts, include beet as an integral part of an anti-cancer diet.**

They're a nutritional powerhouse and available all year round .

Because of their rich color, they are high in antioxidants and phytonutrients, as well as being a great source of Vitamin C and manganese.

Brain health

A recent study found that drinking beet juice improved blood flow to parts of the brain where degeneration from conditions such as Alzheimer's and other forms of cognitive impairment had resulted. The high level of nitrates they contain also produce nitric oxide in the blood which prompts blood vessels to widen and as a result the brain receives more oxygen.

Good for the heart

This natural opening up of blood vessels also means improved heart health. In a study published by the American Heart Association's Hypertension Journal, researchers found that drinking just one glass of beet juice could significantly lower blood pressure within 24 hours.

Beets also have anti-inflammatory properties, meaning they can help with diseases such as diabetes, and they can also assist in the body's natural detox process.

They are also high in fiber which is great news for a healthy gastro-intestinal tract.

My wife, my son and I all use this product daily; I haven't been that excited about a product until now!

Here is my ongoing Healthmasters.com commitment to you: if for any reason you aren't 100% satisfied with this product just call us. No need to return it. Just keep it and please use it. And I will still give you a credit for the full purchase price.

The product is simply that good, plus it's that good for your health. But remember to only use one scoop a day to start with. This product is an incredible liver cleanser. It's really good for your liver as most folks have unhealthy livers.

So let's take this rejuvenating process slowly.

Many of you have eaten a lot of bad stuff. So, now it is time to start on a healthy life style.

This is one of the best and easiest ways to start that journey.

25 | Effective New Protocol that Works to Stop Your Miserable Allergies

Here in Florida, the oak blossoms are creating a tremendous allergy problem. Allergies by the way are easy to control and in most cases eliminated. My allergies were so bad in my 20's that I took 3-5 Sudafed a day. My nick name was Hanky Broer.

Thank God, I finally learned how to get rid of them. This protocol has worked for me and many of my friends and patients over the years.

No pasteurized dairy (except raw organic butter) that means none. Once you get your allergies under control, you can try and reintroduce raw-certified-organic-grass fed dairy. I can use that milk with no allergy response. But in the meantime use Almond milk. We have this available at Health Masters.

Do not use Soy at all ever.

Especially, do not use soy milk and tofu. This is a nasty product that really flares up allergies. Plus, it's loaded with estrogen.

Stop Allergy Protocol. Stop Your Miserable Allergies Now!

Super important use our **GHI Cleanse**. 1 scoop 4x a day. Mix this product in water. It really helps to stop the body's inflammatory response due to allergies. This product is Amazing! Remember allergies and food related intolerance cause a variety of problems.

Problems:		They can also contribute to the following:	
Brain Fog	Bloating	ADHD	Panic Episodes
Sore Joints	Cramping	Depression	Criminal Behavior
Low Energy	Constipation	Confusion	Obsessive Compulsive Behavior
Low Blood Sugar	Diarrhea	Anxiety	Dementia
Heart Irregularities	Unstable PH		

Remember the **story of Alexander C.?** How he was suicidal and had many of the above symptoms. Once we stabilized his inflammatory response and stabilized his blood sugar these symptoms simply disappeared. My family and I went to Alexander's Restaurant this past week. He is doing great. I still speak to him on a regular basis, but because he feels so great and his business has prospered. He doesn't get a chance to come by the house like he used to come by. . I am glad he's doing so well, though I do miss his visits at my home. By the way his wife was hospitalized several weeks ago for low blood pressure and heart irregularities. After extensive testing the medical tests found nothing, imagine that. So they released her and she started on the same program as Alexander and now she feels great. Amazing how it's so easy to help so many and all they have to do is listen.

Next, D3 Again:

Previously, I have written extensive articles on D3. I will again stress how its role in the immune system and allergy control is critical.

By the way, you know I'm not done with soy yet. Let me tell you a few more things about soy. I can't stand this stuff its total and complete poison as far as I am concerned.

- Soy Contains estrogenic compounds.
- One study showed it can alter the development of the male hypothalamus causing males to act like females. Thereby, it can turn little boy's brains into little girl's brains.
- Because the hypothalamus determines sexual behavior, there is a nucleus of the hypothalamus called the "sexual dimorphic nucleus of the preoptic area (SDN-POA)
- When little Boys are fed soy the SDNPOA is reduced in size which can cause problems in learning
- Some studies showed that soy also reduces testosterone
- Some Studies showed that the prostate gland and penis were smaller in men given soy formula as infants

Females given soy showed a reduction in oxytocin (this is called the "love hormone") a decrease in this hormone makes women less interested in sex, and causes a decrease in sexual receptiveness. it also protects the brain form inflammation. As more a more info on soy is revealed along with the science behind it I will bring it to you. For over 30 years I have warned of the dangers of soy. One more thing, exposing a child to soy formula and then subjecting them to the standard vaccination protocol (26 vaccines by age 6) dramatically increased their risk of developing Parkinson's disease as an adult. By the way Soy is also high in fluoride which is a deadly poison. Hopefully you are now starting to understand why I CAN'T STAND THIS PRODUCT. As far as I concerned it should be banned as a farm item.

Here's my anti-inflammatory treatment for inflammation and allergies:

1. No Dairy
2. No Soy
3. **Health Masters GHI Cleanse** More on this below
4. **Health Masters Probiotic Blend** 80% of the immune system involves the gut. It must be taken care of.
5. **Health Masters Excellent C**
6. **Health Masters Ultimate D3** 10,000 IU a day for 30 days then 5000 IU a day. A must for strong immune system
7. **Health Masters Super Potent E with selenium**
8. **Health Masters Ultimate Multiple Vitamin**
9. **Drink Distilled Water** 1/2 your body weight in ounces per day. This is critical; do not ingest chlorine or fluoride. Plus, all the pesticides and chemicals in water.
10. **Health Masters Fermented Cod Liver Oil**

A brief outline of GHI Cleanse

- **G** is for Gut or Gastrointestinal System
- **H** is for Hepatic or Liver function
- **I** is for Inflammation

This product has 26 grams of hypoallergenic pea rice protein (complete protein) It can be used as a meal replacement. It contains all essential Amino Acids it can stop protein malnutrition when used regularly.

- Aminogen Enzyme helps to digest protein
- Over 4000 mgs of glutamine for healthy gut
- Supports all liver pathways for healthy liver function.
- Supports hormone balance and metabolism which begins in the gut and is completed in the liver.
- This is also an incredible anti- aging product. Remember one of the primary causes of aging is inflammation. It basically clears the inflammatory path ways helping to stop all inflammation.
- Its 5 distinctive anti-inflammatory compounds are cumin, ginger bioflavonoid, Rutin, and aniacinameds

I take it every morning before my workout, along with one purple stick (Acai-Energy Boost) and one HGH Stimulate. This 3 part power packed breakfast sends my energy and fat burning metabolism into overdrive. Plus it stops inflammation, helps to reduce the soreness which accompanies proper exercise.

Try this energy drink protocol as soon as you wake up, before you work out. It's Amazing!

Call my office at 1-800-726-1834 to order the supplements recommended above.

26 | Two Steps to Help Avoid Parkinson's Disease

Parkinson's disease is awful. Anyone living with it will attest to the destructive nature of this disease.

It has been a while since I have written on Parkinson's. In the past, I stressed the importance of avoiding pesticides and herbicides. I will now address Parkinson's and solvent exposure.

The dry-cleaning industry today and in years past uses a variety of solvents to clean clothes. Other industries also use these solvents but apparently the latest research on Parkinson's is looking at lifetime exposure to solvents. The solvents which seem to be implicated in Parkinson's are primarily the dry cleaning solvents.

I include in this category:

1. Trichloroethylene
2. Tetrachloroethylene
3. Perchloroethylene

Current studies have shown that when an individual had a six months or greater work related exposure to trichloroethylene that the risk for getting Parkinson's was 6x greater than the unexposed. The other 2 solvents also increased risks. Again these solvents are used in other industries.

I do not know if the wearing of dry cleaned goods can increase the risk. Hopefully, these solvents are rinsed out before the clothes are dried.

Due to toxicity concerns the use of trichloroethylene was supposed to be discontinued in the USA years ago. Due to the huge amount of textile imports from China I believe that China poses a significant health risk to those countries importing from China. I do not know what China uses. They basically have minimal pollution or regulatory controls. When I was there almost 10 years ago the air quality was so bad that almost everyone was wearing a mask and coughing.

What I do know is that Trichloroethylene is one of the primary contaminants of our drinking water. It's detectable in up to 30% of U.S. drinking water. Ground water is filled with it because of the run off of the dry-cleaning industry. This is one of the reasons I have continually pleaded with you for years to only **drink distilled water**. I have been using **distilled water** for over 30 years. Well water is NOT safe in most cases due to ground water contamination.

Plus ALL well water contains dissolved ionic calcium which can contribute to hardening of the arteries.

This new study perfectly fits into my conclusion that Parkinson's is often neurological degeneration due to toxin exposure. Again, please **distill your drinking water**. Imagine that, 30% of drinking water is so contaminated it can cause this disease.

You also might consider taking **Chelation therapy.** While I formulated Chelation therapy to help remove heavy metals, it may help in this area as well.

27 | Healthy Americans Kill Profits for Pharmaceutical Companies

Keeping people sick is big business — very big business — for Big Pharma. After all, sick people buy and refill prescriptions and medications, not healthy ones.

In case you're new to all this, 'Big Pharma' is the nickname given to all of those pharmaceutical companies that act in concert with each other — and not like the separate competing entities as they would have you believe. It is a unique kind of industry in that it controls the entire traditional medical profession, from what's taught in medical schools and what's dispensed to doctors to prescribe their patients, to what health policies our legislators 'approve.' Big Pharma's influence is so firmly entrenched in our doctors' lives that a recurring highlight of most medical careers is the all-expenses paid cruises and 'conferences' to four-star resorts and exotic islands. But let's call these trips what they really are: Brilliantly conceived, well-orchestrated and thinly veiled sales incentives and bribes to push expensive meds on an unsuspecting public. A public that believes their doctor is diagnosing a medical condition based on years of expertise and training — not on the best selling pill du jour. Truth is, your health is in the hands of a corporate executive more concerned about the health of their bottom line than you.

An all too fresh memory of 'doctors burying their mistakes' is the Vioxx debacle.

Before it was finally pulled off the market, Merck & Co.'s arthritis drug Vioxx may have led to more than 27,000 heart attacks and sudden cardiac deaths. According to a 2004 Wall Street Journal article, Merck was aware the drug's health risks and fought hard to keep that news quiet so to protect its $2.5 billion annual blockbuster drug. But clearly that became impossible after an internal study showed that patients taking the drug were more likely to suffer a cardiac event than those taking a placebo.

When it was pulled, two million Americans were taking Vioxx. Even more troubling is now — nearly a decade later — still no one can explain how Vioxx was able to remain on the market as long as it did.

Explaining Which Came First:

Before there was a Big Pharma, people relied on homeopathic or 'alternative' medicine. It was inexpensive, effective and readily purchased from the Sears catalogue. It was also the focus of nearly every medical school in the country.

Then in 1847, explains Dr. Harvey Bigelsen in his eye-opening book, *Medical Conspiracy in America*, the American Medical Association (AMA) — was formed and immediately began defining (dictating, actually) what forms of healing were to be taught and practiced in medical schools. (The association was created with the backing of John D. Rockefeller Sr., oil magnate and the wealthiest man in America.) Homeopathic medicine was now on a collision course with allopathic medicine, which the AMA was aggressively beginning to push on the American public. But the AMA still had a few more tricks up its sleeve: They also put together a commission to investigate and inspect all medical schools — including those in competition with allopathic ones. The Council on Medical Education conducted the survey of 162 medical schools in 1905 and took their finding to Henry S. Pritchett, president of the Carnegie Foundation. Pritchett hired educator Abraham Flexner — whose brother, Simon Flexner, MD, directed all medical research into disease cause and prevention from 1903 through the 1930s at the Rockefeller Institute. It was also decided to tour medical schools in the United States to determine their qualifications to teach. And to fully control the competition, the AMA also established universal licensing boards in all states.

Bigelsen explains further that by 1919, there was a 50 percent reduction in the number of medical school graduates to 2,658. By 1970, there were only 107 medical schools. Only the "good medical schools" (those capable of teaching modern scientific medicine) were financially supported with money from Rockefeller. Homeopathic schools did not use "modern scientific medicine" and did not receive funding from the Rockefeller Foundation and drug companies.

While Abraham Flexner was conducting his study, the AMA created the Propaganda Department, which was headed by Dr. Arthur Cramp, an editorial assistant at the Journal of the American Medical Association (JAMA.).

The committee, comprised of allopathic physicians, reviewed and analyzed various non-allopathic treatments, modalities, and services and reported their unfavorable findings to the council, which published them in JAMA. This anti-competitive activity has been allowed to go on unchecked since it began even though it is a clear violation of the Sherman Antitrust Act.

The introduction of allopathic medicine also meant the birth of pharmacology, the mainstay of organized medicine. Pharmaceuticals required a doctor's prescription, had to be purchased from a pharmacy, and were expensive. What's more, allopathic medicine touted the use of vaccines that often contained lethal amounts of active disease agents in the serum, which could result in death of the patient. Homeopathic remedies? Little or no risk? Period.

The Centers for Disease Control (CDC) reports thousands of deaths each year directly linked to deadly reactions to such vaccines. What's more, they state, "Allopathic doctors are not trained in nutrition nor are they trained to see the connection between many degenerative diseases and prolonged clinical malnutrition. Instead, allopathic doctors are taught the proper sanctioned surgical or sanctioned pharmaceutical treatment. As often as not, these surgical and pharmaceutical treatments are ineffective or only mask symptoms, but do not cure or alleviate the root problem or ailment. Pharmaceutical treatments do however generate massive profits for pharmaceutical companies and the allopathic doctors who are the only sanctioned pushers of the sanctioned drugs. This situation is no accident."

It is also no accident that hundreds of 'qualified' physicians are overprescribing meds and burying their mistakes. As I stated earlier in this chapter, keeping people sick continues the long-established tradition and goal of Big Pharma — to keep making massive amounts of money.

But here's what really surprised me: Rockefeller himself had a personal preference for homeopathy and died at the age of 97 with his personal homeopathic physician, Dr. H. L. Merryday of Daytona Beach, Florida, in attendance. Imagine, the man who formed the medical industry did not use it Rockefelle,r in my opinion, saw allopathic medicine as simply a way to take money he made from Standard Oil and use it to make even more money via the pharmaceutical industry Keeping you sick is big business! Whether most doctors realize it or not, wellness is not, and never has been, the goal of allopathic medicine.

According to, Karl Loren, author of *The New Medical Monopoly — Allopathy*, "Single-handedly, John D. Rockefeller Sr. destroyed the prevailing medical model and created the new one—allopathic medicine. The primary result of this activity was that his crude oil, worth perhaps a nickel per gallon, suddenly, turned into medical drugs, worth hundreds of dollars per gallon."

Backed by Rockefeller money, even then allopathic medicine was a runaway money train.

BIG PHARMA, CORRUPTING EVERYONE IN SIGHT

Just how influential has Big Pharma been on legislation? It's pretty well known that the pharmaceutical manufacturing industry has had one of the largest lobbying efforts on Capitol Hill for years. Here's how it breaks down: With its 1,274 registered lobbyists in Washington D.C., the top 20 pharmaceutical companies and their two trade groups, Pharmaceutical Research and Manufacturers of America (PhRMA) and Biotechnology Industry Organization, lobbied on at least 1,600 pieces of legislation between 1998 and 2004. The non-partisan Center for Responsive Politics says that pharmaceutical companies spent $900 million on lobbying between 1998 and 2005 — more than any other industry. During the same period, they donated $89.9 million to federal candidates and political parties, giving approximately three times as much to Republicans as to Democrats. According to the Center for Public Integrity, from January 2005 through June 2006 alone, the pharmaceutical industry spent approximately $182 million on Federal lobbying.

In 2010 the Center for
Responsible Politics had this to add:

"The pharmaceutical manufacturing industry will likely fair better this decade now that President Barack Obama's initial plan to institute a public health insurance did not become a part of sweeping health care reform legislation signed into law in 2010. A government-run plan, because of its size, would have had considerable negotiating power to draw down drug prices.

Pharmaceutical companies scored major victories during the period President George W. Bush occupied office. In 2003, Bush signed legislation that created Medicare "Part D," expanding benefits to include prescription drugs. However, the bill prevents the government from negotiating prices with drug companies."

What's even more disturbing is the leaked 2009 White House memo, which details of the deal President Obama made with Big Pharma.

The memo — obtained by The Huffington Post — was first denied by the White House and Big Pharma reps, then later confirmed by the New York Times, was prepared by a person directly involved in the negotiations, and lists exactly what the White House gave up, and what it got in return.

It says the White House agreed to oppose any congressional efforts to use the government's leverage to bargain for lower drug prices or import drugs from Canada — and also agreed not to pursue Medicare rebates or shift some drugs from Medicare Part B to Medicare Part D, which would cost Big Pharma billions in reduced reimbursements.

In exchange, the Pharmaceutical Researchers and Manufacturers Association (PhRMA) agreed to cut $80 billion in projected costs to taxpayers and senior citizens over ten years. Or, as the memo says: "Commitment of up to $80 billion, but not more than $80 billion."

By the way, the ban on negotiating for lower drug prices was led through Congress in 2003 by then-Louisiana Representative Billy Tauzin, later the president and CEO of PhRMA. As head of PhRMA, Tauzin was a key player in 2009 health care reform negotiations. In 2010 he received $11.6 million from PhRMA, making him the highest-paid health-law lobbyist.

I think this memo puts to bed any lingering question of whether or not the White House and our elected officials are in the pocket of Big Pharma.

28 | Eradication of the Sick and Elderly

The control over what medical plans cover, how much treatment is allowed the elderly and even limitations to the power of doctors forms the basis of Obamacare. One of the authors of this policy is former U.S. Senator and former U.S. Senate Majority Leader Tom Daschle. In his book, *Critical: What We Can Do About the Healthcare Crisis*, what he writes reads like a death sentence on the elderly: One, that seniors be categorically denied treatment so that resources can be spent on the young and the able, and two, that seniors who receive a "hopeless diagnosis" should accept their condition and not seek treatment for it.

Shocking, absolutely! But, I've saved the best for last.

In 2009 Dr. Ezekiel Emanuel, the brother of Rahm Emmanuel, the President's former Chief of Staff and now Mayor of Chicago, was a special advisor (if not the top advisor!) to President Obama on health care.

He famously published an article in which he stated that doctors take the Hippocratic Oath too seriously, and that he advocates denying care to the elderly and disabled.

He says care should not be based on individualism, but on communitarianism. He also believed that the government should be the ones in control of every facet of health, and that the costs of healthcare should be spent on those that will be productive within the community, primarily those between the ages of 15 and 40. Those with disabilities should not be given the same level of treatment, nor should the elderly.

"Suppose a 25-year-old and a 65-year-old have a life threatening disease. Since the 25-year-old has many more potential years of life ahead of him, he should receive preferential treatment."

This is how he justified his thoughts. "The complete lives system discriminates against older people . . . Unlike allocation by sex or race, allocation by age is not invidious discrimination; every person lives through different life stages rather than being a single age. Even if 25-year-olds receive priority over 65-year-olds, everyone who is 65 years now was previously 25 years."

In a separate article written more than 10 years ago for the influential " Hastings Center Report," Emanuel said health services should not be guaranteed to "individuals who are irreversibly prevented from being or becoming participating citizens." He continued, "An obvious example is not guaranteeing health services to patients with dementia."

In a classic case of backpedaling, Emanuel now claims his words were taken out of context. But those words have prompted at least a historian and several politicians alike to label him as a "Deadly Doctor" and denounce his philosophy as "downright evil."

WHY ARE WE GIVING OUR CHILDREN SCHEDULE 2 DRUGS?

Many of you who know me, know that this has been one of my primary topics for over 20 years. Dr. Leon Eisenberg, the founder of the diagnosis ADHD or should I say the inventor of the disease in 1968, died in 2012. But not before he was interviewed by the German magazine, *Der Spiegel* in which he confessed that he made up the disease. I guess he must have had a moment of clarity and conscience to admit he made it up. I am diametrically opposed to Ritalin, a schedule 2 drug in the same category as morphine, as a first treatment protocol especially for a "made up" disease. Ritalin is simply overprescribed.

If you had any question of the abuse of Ritalin in this country, consider this: The U.S. uses 90% of the world's Ritalin. And, from 2007 to 2012, sales of stimulants to treat attention deficit hyperactivity disorder (ADHD) more than doubled from $4 billion to $9 billion, according to a report in the New York Times (March 31, 2013).

That dramatic spike in sales is stoking fears that the drugs are being prescribed not merely to treat ADHD, but to enhance performance in school, improve falling grades or just to keep fidgety kids from disturbing classrooms. Fueling this prescription writing frenzy, says the CDC, is the fact more doctors are diagnosing a growing number of kids as having ADHD. Currently, nearly one in five high school age boys and 11 percent of school-age children overall have been labeled with the diagnosis. In a 2013 interview with the New York Times, CDC director Dr. Thomas R. Frieden, allowed how 'the right medications for ADHD, given to the right people, can make a huge difference.' "Unfortunately, misuse appears to be growing at an alarming rate."

The CDC survey completed in 2012 found an estimated 6.4 million children ages 4 to 17 had been diagnosed at some point, a 53 percent increase over the past decade. Approximately two-thirds of those currently diagnosed have been prescribed drugs such as Ritalin or Aderol. And while those drugs can help patients with ADHD, they can also cause addiction, anxiety and psychosis.

What's surprising is that this increase in new diagnosis comes just 15 years after a national scandal practically erupted regarding the over-prescription of Ritalin and similar drugs to millions of diagnosed children. (I wonder if we, as a culture, have shorter memories or if the drug makers just got more creative in their marketing.)

What's being prescribed these days seems to include everything from Ritalin, Adderall and Adderall XR, Concerta, Focalin and Focalin XR, Metadate CD and Metadate ER, Ritalin SR, Ritalin LA, Elavil, Norpramin, Tofranil or other tricyclic antidepressants, Catapres and Wellbutrin. There was even talk about children receiving Risperdal, an anti-psychotic drug with a bit of a history. According to Dr. David Healy, an internationally respected psychiatrist, psychopharmacologist, scientist, author and professor of psychiatry in Wales, Risperdal was used in the Soviet Union to extract information from political prisoners. "When you think about giving (those drugs) to kids, it's a whole new ball game."

It's actually more than a new ball game — it's a game changer. As reported in the Journal of the American Academy of Child & Adolescent Psychiatry (January 2010), kids as young as two have received this and other drugs for their 'problems'. Predictably, the drugs have an effect on the kids not unlike amphetamines and cocaine.

But who or what is behind this movement to stuff kids with all kinds of pharmaceuticals?... And, I ask why?

The pharmaceutical companies, of course! A lifetime of "just reach for a pill to solve a problem (real or imagine)" is a very profitable way to make a living, generation after generation. Investors have a word for this. Perpetuity: It means 'for life' and it's how they make money on an investment, even after the initial investment has been paid back.

It's believed that Big Pharma does something similar. Because they make truckloads of money from sickness and misery, it makes sense that they would have to keep a few illnesses and diseases in the pipeline . . . so they could pitch a newly developed (and expensive) pill to doctors, describe what it does in carefully worded commercials, entice desperate patients to request it and deliver to stakeholders another year of record profits. And of course, the condition they invent has to have a name with a nice, scary ring to it.

There are many who believe that ADHD is just that — a nonexistent condition discovered during a marketing meeting and then endorsed by Dr. Eisenberg, and others who are convinced that ADHD is the catalyst to triggering long-term child drug abuse. . Some believe that Big Pharma is actively working on convincing people that there's even something called 'adult ADHD.'

Adults having problems are being told they may have adult ADHA and are being offered drugs for it. Pharmaceutical companies market these drugs aggressively. How can General Practitioners refuse to prescribe a drug "proven to work?"

One of the most heartbreaking examples of a drug company addressing an illness that didn't necessarily require a pharmaceutical treatment was the global tragedy involving a morning sickness relief drug called thalidomide.

Developed in the late 1950s, thalidomide was popular in Europe as a sedative and antiemetic for elderly patients. Although neither tested nor approved for use during pregnancy, the effectiveness and absence of significant side-effects led many physicians to prescribe it to pregnant women. Before long it was available over-the-counter. Then the problems began surfacing. Soon afterwards, between 5,000 and 7,000 infants were born with malformation of the limbs, called phocomelia. Only 40 percent of these children survived.

It was quickly discovered that 50 percent of the mothers with deformed children had taken thalidomide during the first trimester of pregnancy. Throughout Europe and Australia 10,000 cases were reported of infants with phocomelia; with only half of them surviving. Other birth defects included: deformed eyes, hearts, alimentary, and urinary tracts, and blindness and deafness.

Sadly, this example is only one of a plethora of examples I could use. The simple truth is this when it comes to Big Pharma, It is always about the money. Period!

29 | A Prostate Supplement That Works

Are you one of the millions of men concerned enough about your prostate health, that you're actually doing something about it? Are you taking a prostate supplement because you need to? And are you following the manufacturers' direction and taking so many at one time, you find yourself gagging before the sixth, seventh and eighth pill is finally down? And have you ever wondered why these health supplements are always 'horse pills'? You know the ones . . . they're available in just two sizes — Shetland and Clydesdale!

Guys, listen . . . there's a better way! I'm here to tell you there's something easier to ingest and something you'll actually look forward to taking. And here's the best part: It really works!! So say good-bye to trace amounts of dozens of ingredients. Say goodbye to soy and other toxic fillers. Say goodbye to expensive, inflated costly solutions. And say 'hello' to the prostate breakthrough you've been waiting for. at a price that'll make you smile.

HEALTHY PROSTATE 101:

There isn't a guy on the planet who doesn't want a healthy prostate. In fact, most of us have heard the horror stories of what it's like to live with an enlarged prostate . . . stories which begin and end with the words 'painful' and 'suffering' and 'waking up every couple of hours in the middle of the night to run to the bathroom.' So what are your options? You could take a prescription medication called alpha-blockers like Flomax, Hytrin, Rapaflo, or Proscar. But . . . these meds don't work for everyone and the documented side effects which occur with long-term use are very, very scary. Or you can continue reading this to find out about an awesome, natural alternative that I recently came across. It's been an incredibly popular remedy, globally, for dealing with benign prostatic hyperplasia (BPH), a common prostate condition that affects many men after the age of 50.

The symptoms include frequent nighttime urination and the inability to completely empty the bladder. It may be common, but it's still pretty unpleasant. And you don't want it happening to you. (This is the same product that worked so well with my cousin Fritz in Germany).

Let me tell you another story . . . Several years ago I had a well- known pastor visit me in Florida. I noticed over the course of his visit he had to use the bathroom every 30 minutes or so. He told me though he'd had this problem for a while and it had been getting worse. At that time he was only in his 30's — way too young to be suffering from a prostate problem. Without thinking twice about it, I handed him eight Health Masters' Prostate Support tablets, instructing him to take four now and the remaining four the next day.

Guess what? By the third day he was no longer running to the bathroom every few minutes. Frequent urination . . . gone! This natural supplement takes care of that problem it in most cases. And what is that popular natural alternative? It's a powerhouse compound combination called Pygeum Extract and Uva-Ursi Extract. This combination contains beta-sitosterol -- a naturally occurring phytosterol found in low concentrations in many of the fruits and vegetables that form part of a healthy diet. To these two ingredients we also add saw palmetto, pygeum africanum, and pumpkin seeds to help with various prostate problems. And what makes them so effective? You guessed it -- beta-sitosterol.

This easily tops my list of the most exciting modern breakthroughs in prostate support. You know I don't get easily excited over every new product that comes down the pike. Because I'm a scientist and researcher, I'm skeptical and methodical. I need to see the research. And I need to believe that research before I go any further. I'm here to tell you that I saw the research and my skepticism melted away like butter in a microwave.

Listen to this . . . Over the past few years, several well-controlled scientific studies of the beneficial effects of beta-sitosterol on prostate problems have been published in reputable journals. Most of these studies have dealt with the use of beta-sitosterol in controlling the troublesome problems of an enlarged prostate. In 1995, a randomized, double-blind, placebo-controlled multicenter trial published in the British journal, The Lancet, studied 200 men who suffered from BPH. After six months, the study concluded that: "Significant improvement in symptoms and urinary flow parameters show the effectiveness of beta-sitosterol in the treatment of BPH."

A similar study, published by the British Journal of Urology in 1997, studied another 177 BPH sufferers, again for six months. These results showed that: "There were significant improvements over placebo in those treated with beta-sitosterol." This led the authors to conclude that "Beta-sitosterol is an effective option in the treatment of BPH."

Then, two years later, a U.S.-based review was conducted of all well-controlled studies of the use of beta-sitosterol in the treatment of BPH. Four separate studies that passed the authors' stringent criteria were identified. Of these, an overall total of 519 men suffering from mild to moderate BPH were studied. Although the authors commented that the studies were too short-term and that there was a lack of standardization of preparation of beta-sitosterol, they concluded that for sufferers of BPH: "Beta-sitosterol improves urological symptoms and flow measures." I like when studies conclude with words like . . . 'significant improvement' . . . 'effective option' . . . 'improves symptoms'.

Those words are music to a research scientist's ears like mine. Words like that also mean I can offer a product to my friends and clients good enough to be part of the Health Masters family of superior quality supplements. Simply put: You'll wake up refreshed and alert and be better at your job because you've been able to sleep through the night . . . You'll never have to choke down a bunch of horse pills again . . . Actually, you take just two small soft gels a day that's been proven to be effective — without the side effects of an expensive prescription medication . . . and without costing you a king's ransom. You'll be able to completely drain your bladder in most cases . . . And you'll hopefully once again have a powerful urine stream without pain (that alone is worth the price of admission!) . . . and speaking of price, the days of paying through the nose for a healthy prostate are OVER!

SAVE MONEY AND GET MORE
OF THE GOOD STUFF:

Don't you wish everything was like that? Now if you're wondering where saw palmetto is in all of this, I'll tell you. The top quality saw palmetto is at times, difficult to come by and consequently, expensive. (Unfortunately, some less than ethical manufacturers cheat the public by including inferior product in their formulations — which ultimately does nothing for you.) My formulation always, only uses the highest quality source of saw palmetto, pygeum and pumpkin seed. (Note: I should also mention that beta-sisterol has a chemical structure similar to healthy cholesterol.)

So here's the bottom line: I have a superior natural alternative that I'm pleased with and I know works. Need more to convince you? Try this: This healthy prostate powerhouse I've been talking about . . . is at a price that won't rival your cable bill. I know you're liking that! And . . . it's so effective, you can actually visit your doctor when you want to instead of when it's a prostate-related emergency. That means now you can have something powerful enough to actually keep your prostate healthy at every stage of your life!

And the name of this healthy prostate powerhouse? Health Masters' Prostate Support

My friends and clients have been asking me to recommend a healthy prostate supplement for a very long time that also ensures that they'll be able to perform at their peak when it matters most. Health Masters' Prostate Support is what I'll be recommending — not only for the benefits of beta-sitosterol, but also for the powerful nutrients I've added to support, boost and maintain prostate health.

So, what are those nutrients?

Zinc (**Health Masters' Zinc Glycinate**) Zinc is critical to men's health and all aspects of male reproduction, including hormone metabolism and balance, prostate function, and sperm formation and motility. Yet, more than 70% of men don't get the minimum daily requirement of zinc from their diets. Zinc is one of the most important supplements for men's health with the highest concentrations in the prostate gland. It is a key mineral in male sexual function and a protector nutrient against prostate cancer. Zinc also maximizes your testosterone production. In fact, low testosterone and low sperm counts may be signs of a zinc deficiency.

Health Masters' Prostate Support supplies a 15 mg of zinc in an easy-to-absorb form. I have been taking zinc for over 30 years. It also has the added benefit of increasing libido in many men, Vitamin B6 (**Health Masters' Corticare B5 B6**) Vitamin B6 has long been recognized as an important vitamin to maintain prostate health. The Linus Pauling Institute says that vitamin B6 can stop cycles of inflammation in the prostate and be useful in lowering levels of prolactin in the body. Elevated prolactin is linked with erectile dysfunction and reproductive health challenges. Optimal prolactin levels can ensure healthy sexual function and help control levels of prostate enlargement.

In fact, a recent Swedish study from the American Journal of Clinical Nutrition suggests that men with earlier-stage prostate cancer may have better survival odds if they get a bit more than the recommended amount of vitamin B6 every day. The recommended dosage of B6 for men age 50 and younger is 1.3 mg daily, while older men are encouraged to get 1.7 mg The men in the Swedish study averaged 2.2 to 2.9 mg per day. The protective effect of B6 appeared to help men whose tumors had not yet spread beyond the prostate at the time of diagnosis. Vitamin B6 is found in a range of foods, including beans, potatoes, bananas, meat, chicken, peanut butter and certain fish, namely salmon.

Health Masters' Prostate Support is packed with 5 mg of prostate-boosting vitamin B6. All the healthy prostate defense AND support you could possibly want . . . in just two small soft gel caplets. And, the best part of this top quality, dependable support is that costs just pennies a day. Join the men doing something remarkable for themselves and their families — as they protect the health of their prostates and take Health Masters' Prostate Support. No more waking up to run to the bathroom several times in the middle of the night. No more choking down multiple horse pills. No more expensive supplements that rival the cost of your cable bill. No more wondering if your prostate support supplement is really doing what it's supposed to do. Save your cash. Save your prostate. It's all here. A proven and reliable prostate remedy: Two softgel caplets for less than 75 cents a day. It's time to take control and discover what Health Masters has to offer.

30 | Simple Remedy for Joint and Back Pain

The term osteoporosis literally means porous bones. This problem occurs more dramatically in women, with at least 1.2 million American women over age 45 suffering bone fractures from osteoporosis each year. Both men and women suffer from this disease and of these, hundreds of thousands of them die within one year from complications arising from these fractures. Many of the survivors of hip fractures and hip replacement surgeries will remain permanently disabled! A decreased level of absorbable calcium in the blood is the primary cause of osteoporosis.

What is arthritis and osteoporosis?

What is the natural remedy? Get back your mobility and arthritis pain relief without taking life threatening drugs. Why osteoporosis was an unknown disease 60 years ago. What you and your family are eating that dissolves calcium from your bones?

Let me explain why this disease did not exist in our grandparent's day, and why the foods you eat can cause this debilitating disease. Calcium has to be digested in your stomach and absorbed into your bloodstream to be absorbed into your bones.

Women and men alike are taking calcium supplements like never before in this country, yet in a study done by the American Journal of Public Health, it shows that there are more hip fractures from women that drink pasteurized, homogenized processed milk. Why are these women not absorbing the calcium in the milk they are drinking? Why are their bones de-calcifying?

There are two reasons for the de-calcification of our bones. The first is that by the time you reach the age of 50, your stomach has dramatically reduced the amount of acid it needs to breakdown the calcium. When it doesn't breakdown the calcium in the stomach, it then passes through the body without ever making it to our organs and cells for absorption. Your calcium isn't by itself, this also happens to all of your vital nutrients. This, by the way is easily corrected by using our **Digestive Enzyme Blend**. I highly recommend this product. It helps the body to digest food and get better absorption than any product I have ever used. It is important for those approaching 40 and an absolute necessity if you are over 50. I take 4 with each meal.

The second culprit keeping your body from absorbing your calcium is excess phosphorus in your diet. Since the 1950's phosphorus has been added to our food supply at increasing amounts as time goes on. Phosphorus will counteract any calcium you are taking by supplementation or in your food supply. The foods that contain the most of this decalcifying substance that causes your bones to be brittle and weak are carbonated soft drinks (phosphoric acid), processed foods, caffeine, high protein, and sugar consumption. Most people 50-60 years ago were not eating a high phosphorus diet. Most of them drank unprocessed raw cow's milk full of rich absorbable natural enzyme loaded calcium.

Many of you have seen a skeleton hanging in a science lab or doctor's office, this is not a true representation of bone. Believe it or not, bones are actually living. If you do not believe me, just ask anyone who broke one. They bleed, produce pain, and repair just like any other part of the body. And, they need proper nutrition just as much as any other part of the body to do this. Without a doubt, dietary factors, such as non-absorbable calcium, insufficient hydrochloric acid and digestive enzymes, and a lack of resistance exercise contribute significantly to increasing bone loss in men and women alike.

This disease can in many cases be corrected by making the dietary changes and lifestyle changes offered in our program, *Maximum Energy Health & Fitness*, and by following our supplement plan. All supplements are not created equal! If you are looking for the solution, you must take the right supplements and make healthy lifestyle changes. Some of the recommended supplements to reverse bone loss are **Regeneration, Ossomag, Ultimate D3-5000, Digestive Enzyme Blend, Ultimate Multiple** and our **Cod Liver Oil**. Please call our office at 1-800-726-1834, if you have questions about this or the products. Either myself, or one of my well-trained staff will be happy to help you with your questions. Or visit our website Healthmasters.com

Now let's talk about Arthritis, and its causes and cures: Many people are not aware that Osteoporosis and Osteoarthritis are very closely associated. Arthritis afflicts more than 30 million Americans and can result in severe pain and restrictions in daily activities for those who suffer its ravages. There are actually several forms of arthritis, with osteoarthritis being by far the most common type. Osteoarthritis is different from rheumatoid arthritis, which is a disease process where the body's own immune cells attack and destroy the linings of the joint cavities in the body. Osteoarthritis is more of a wear-and-tear kind of degeneration.

Osteoarthritis is also known as degenerative joint disease. It appears to be associated with certain types of occupations, previous injuries, family tendency, and especially to being overweight. It is characterized by an inflammation, breakdown, and eventual loss of the cartilage between the joints. Normally, a thin layer of cartilage covers the ends of the bones in a joint. This cartilage acts as a cushion or shock absorber to prevent the bones of the joint from rubbing together during movement. There is also a very thick, very slippery mucus-like liquid between these joints called synovial fluid, which acts as a lubricant. Synovial fluid is produced by an organ called the bursae. Inflammation or infection in these bursae is called bursitis, and should not be confused with any form of arthritis.

Remember Vioxx? Millions of Vioxx pills were taken before the public found out the death rates associated with this product. If you remember the talk show you originally heard me on, I have been warning people all over the country about the dangers of Vioxx and other cox 2 arthritis drugs for years before they were taken off the market.

To those of you who listened to me, you didn't become one of the 140,000 cases of heart disease and death reported to the Congress by the FDA whistle blower. It is quite simple, you can't rely on the FDA for the truth. Recently I did a radio show out of New York. When I made this statement the hosts were shocked! The next question was, do have anything to back up that claim? I simply gave them the facts, 50% of the drugs approved by the FDA are removed from the market or have their warnings changed within 5 years. Also remember, that I warned everyone 15 years ago that Prozac and Zoloft increased suicide rates in children. The medical and research and drug company folks really got mad about that one! Yet the FDA now requires a black box warning on these drugs for potential suicide in children.

Quite frankly we simply can't rely on the FDA to protect any of us from dangerous drugs. Perfect example, why are cigarettes still sold in the United States? Enough said.

While all these cover-ups and mass poisonings are going on, the FDA, pharmaceutical companies and many doctors continue to ridicule natural treatments, supplementation and proper diet and exercise.

The reality is this, there are in many cases, inexpensive and extremely effective ways to solve health problems without relying on life threatening, overly promoted miracle drugs. Let me give you a personal example. Several months ago, I had a back injury. I was having tremendous pain in my hip and left leg. Sitting was excruciatingly painful. But I knew there was a natural treatment. I dug deep into the literature and guess what? I found the solution; I am now pain free and drug free. WOW!

Remember many people only get relief from the terrible pain of Arthritis and back pain by taking NSAID's, (non-steroidal anti-inflammatory drug). These are very dangerous drugs and have as I have already mentioned, have many life threatening side effects. The recent bad news of these drugs has left a lot of people without a way to manage the day-to-day pain of this debilitating disease.

Here are the alternatives I have found that workextremely well with the day-to-day stiffness of Arthritis, back pain, and they also help to replace bone loss.

H~G~H Stimulate	Improves circulatory, immune and nervous system function, memory, reduces wrinkles, increases bone density, and decreases blood pressure.++
Ultimate Multiple	Gives foundation nutrition for wellness and disease protection.
Ultimate D3-5000	Super dose vitamin D. A must for anyone with osteoporosis/osteopenia.
Cod Liver Oil	Our High-Vitamin Pure Cod Liver Oil, offers more vitamin A and D than any other product on the market.
GHI Cleanse	Used to treat chronic inflammatory conditions. We use this product daily, it's incredible!
Salicin	Offers anti-inflammatory properties, pain relief and antioxidant support. A natural pain reliever safe to use for extended periods.
Regeneration	Helps to build strong bones, hair and nails
Joint Support	Rebuilds joint, cartilage and connective tissue.
Ossomag	Superior calcium, magnesium and D3 formula to reduce and replace bone loss
Cortico B5-B6	Offers water-soluble B vitamins to insure strong bones, balance and mobility.
Aqua Trace	Trace minerals to support joints, connective tissue and strong bones.
Excellent C	Helps protect and support healthy connective tissue.
Digestive Enzyme Blend	Imperative to breaking down calcium and nutrients for absorption.
Adrenal Support	Helps to restore adrenals and reduces cortisol the stress hormone that makes you store body fat. This one also increases energy levels.
Super Potent E	Excellent for heart, circulation and cancer prevention.
B Complex	Important for the support of the adrenal hormone production, regulation of the body's production of energy through enhancement of Coenzyme A production.

Also remember to reduce or eliminate the nightshade variety of vegetables. They include tomatoes, eggplant, bell peppers and white potatoes. They can inflame your joints.

31 | Specific Details on Some of Our Products

Health Masters Ultimate Multiple:

I always try to provide you with the best products possible. They are the same products that my family and I use every day. Remember these facts, never use tablet vitamins if at all possible. There is so much glue and heat used in producing these products it is literally impossible for your body to break them down. They go right through your body unused. Secondly don't use gelatin capsules use only cellulose fiber capsules. Gelatin capsules are probably pork by product. Less than 1% of all products use cellulose fiber capsules because of the cost. They are much more expensive than tablets or gelatin capsules. All of my Health Masters products use only cellulose capsules. Plus my multiple uses only activated B vitamins. Most cheap vitamins use cyancobil amine this is a cyanide B-12 vitamin and is very toxic. The body cannot use it. It is poison. Our B-12 is methyl cobal amine, which is highly absorbable. A lot of times cheap products will list their B-12 as cobal amine. They won't tell you whether it's methyl cobal amine, or cyancobil amine, guess why? It's because they use the cheap cyancobil amine and they don't want you to know their product is toxic. Our B-12 is 10 times more expensive than the poisonous one. But our product works. We carry the best products period. Our multiple also has 200 IU of natural E. 99% of all grocery store vitamins use useless synthetic E. Our multiple is also patented to release energy by containing Vanadium, Chromium, and Biotin which are critical ingredients for energy production and fat burning. Our product really helps you to feel better. I take it every day. The dosing is to take 2 twice a day.

Excellent C:

This is a functional vitamin C formula. It has added 7.5 mg of Bioperine per capsule. Bioperine is a proprietary, patented piperine extract that has been shown in clinical studies to increase the bio-availability of vitamin C by up to 40%. Vitamin C provides valuable anti-oxidant protection and supports the production of collagen and healthy connective tissue. Excellent C is buffered to help prevent potential stomach upset often found with high dietary ascorbic acid intake.

Super Potent E:

This is a mixed tocopheral product, which is high in gamma E. This is the most potent E to protect against LDL cholesterol (the bad one) breakdown. When you oxidize or breakdown the LDL cholesterol it's like turning little razor blades loose in your arteries. This oxidized LDL cholesterol actually creates lesions (little cuts) in the blood vessels. These little cuts then form scars, which can cause blockages in the arteries, heart disease and heart attacks. I recommend 1600 IU for men and 800 IU for women daily. By the way, I have been taking 1600 IU for 25 years. The study several years ago saying E was bad used chemically produced cheap synthetic E. No study has ever shown that natural mixed tocopheral E does anything but good.

Cortico B5-B6:

This supplement supplies significant amounts of water- soluble B vitamins. They are important for the support of the adrenal hormone production, regulation and the body's own production of energy through its enhancement of Coenzyme A production. Activated B vitamins are utilized in this formula for optimal effectiveness.

Adrenal Support:

Clinical Applications

- Stress Reduction During the "Alarm" & "Exhaustive" Phases
- Adaptation to Stress (caused by temperature changes, sleep deprivation, negative emotions, physical exertion, trauma or illness.)
- Immune Support
- Antioxidant/Cyto protection

Adrenal Support is a comprehensive blend of standardized extracts of highest quality adaptogenic herbs and three relevant B vitamins. These ingredients support the body's stress response by aiding in adrenal hormone production and assisting in stress adaptation. The formula is designed to reduce stress-induced fatigue and exhaustion, protect tissues from free radicals and may aid in simulating the body's immune system.

Cordyceps sinensis is a safe, highly valued, adapting herb with pharmacological activities proven to benefit nearly every physiological system that is affected by stress, including the immune system and cardiovascular system (e.g. prevention of heart arrhythmia's, platelet aggregation and clot formation). It has a positive effect upon blood sugar, cholesterol and tryglycerides levels. Cordyceps has been employed for dizziness, weakness and general wasting and is used to reduce fatigue, increase energy and enhance stamina. The herb has documented antioxidant activity.

Rhodiola rosea Root has been traditionally used to increase stamina and reduce fatigue, depression, nervous disorders, infections and impotence. Russian researchers demonstrated the root counteracted mental and physical fatigue and a host of stressors. The root extract may be able to prevent stress-induced cardiac damage and may be anti-arrhythmic. Research has shown that Rhodiola rosea has an effect on brain neurotransmitters such as dopamine and serotonin and might increase engogenous opioids.

Panax ginseng helps to restore adrenals. In stress, Panax ginseng reduced ulcers and reversed elevated blood sugar. Ginsenosides have pain relieving and anti-inflammatory activities. It also reduces cortisol, the stress hormone which makes you store body fat.

Vitamin B6 and Pantothenic Acid assist in protecting the body from the ravages of stress including related fatigue. Pantothenic acid is essential to the adrenal glands for production of the glucocorticoids. It forms pantethine in the body that then converts to Coenzyme A. D-Calcium pantothenate contains 91.96% pantothenic acid and is the usual supplemental form. Vitamin B6, acting as a co-enzyme, has a role in the conversion of muscle sugar to glucose needed for the stress response, is involved with synthesis of serotonin and enhances the immune system.

Please enjoy this testimony from Diana Yoder.

Dr Broer,

You may not remember, my name is Diana Yoder from Pastor Rod Parsley's church.(We did a TV interview with Pastor Rod Parsley 2 and half years ago). I was diagnosed with Graves Disease 6 months prior to our meeting. I have been on your *Eat, Drink and Be Healthy* program and lots of your vitamins and supplements and I have had a clean bill of health every check up since. The doctor keeps telling me everything is Bulls eye perfect. cholesterol, blood pressure, triglycerides. I am 54 years old and feel great!!! I am now taking the **H•G•H Stimulate** and love it!! I was just told today by someone, "I don't know what you are doing but you look so young." I have not been sick a day in those 2 and half years since starting your program and taking your vitamins and supplements.

Thanks and God Bless You,

Diana Yoder

All of these high quality supplements can also be purchased by calling my office at 1-800-726-1834.

32 | Say No to Gas, Bloating, and Indigestion

Struggling with acid reflux and heartburn is a nuisance and inhibits living life to the fullest.

Say NO to them today and enjoy this simple remedy:

Acid Reflux and Heartburn:

To clean up digestion problems try the following:

At the beginning of a meal or within the first five minutes of starting a meal:

DIGESTIVE ENZYME BLEND
- If you eat a light meal — take 1
- If you eat a medium meal — take 2
- If you eat a heavy meal — take 3
AFTER EVERY MEAL

GASTRAGEST
- If you eat a light meal — take 1
- If you eat a medium meal — take 2
- If you eat a heavy meal — take 3
AND

IMMUNE SUPPORT DF
- Take 8 capsules throughout the day maybe 4 in the AM and 4 in the PM. If you are not going to take 8 a day, don't take any.

Continue doing this until the digestion is cleared up!

I also highly recommend following my *Eat Drink and Be Healthy* series.

You will find more information online about our powerful Immune Support DF at Healthmasters. Com.

33 | Discovery for Diabetics

In this world of throwing drugs at symptoms and hoping for the best, there is a growing number of health experts who are shouting, "There's a better way!" Even if the medical community won't listen, I'm hoping you will. You see, the problem with many drugs is the harmful side effects that accompany them. You treat one problem and create three others. That's definitely the case when it comes to treating type-2 diabetes with insulin. If I were to tell you that treating type-2 diabetes with insulin is more dangerous than not treating it all, would you believe me? Sometimes the cure can be worse than the actual disease.

In a study that involved 84,622 primary care patients with type-2 diabetes, researchers divided the patients into three groups: sulfonylurea therapy only, insulin therapy only and insulin plus Metformin. Then, the researchers followed these patients to see which events happened first or at all—a cardiac event, cancer or death. They also monitored for microvascular disease. Here's what they discovered. The group that used insulin suffered more heart mortality, more stroke morbidity, more renal complications and neuropathy and more cancer!

Bottom line, insulin is the hormone of aging and death. So, why use it when there are healthier alternatives? Many type-2 diabetics are able to eradicate diabetes with a healthy diet, lifestyle and supplements—no drugs at all. And, instead of having negative side effects like insulin, the healthier way of living also fixes their high cholesterol, triglycerides, hypertension and many more health issues.

TURMERIC EXTRACT PROVES HELPFUL FOR PRE-DIABETIC PATIENTS

Here's some good news. *The Journal of the American Diabetes Association* recently declared that turmeric extract is 100 percent successful at preventing pre-diabetic patients from becoming full-blown diabetic patients over the course of a nine-month turmeric intervention. The study's primary focus was to assess the effectiveness of curcumin in turmeric as a type of delaying agent of type 2 diabetes mellitus (T2DM).

The study was designed as a randomized, double-blinded, placebo-controlled trial of 240 people who were considered prediabetics according to the criteria set by the American Diabetic Association. All subjects were randomly given either 250 mg of curcuminoid or placebo capsules for nine months. Throughout those nine months, the researchers assessed the type 2 diabetes progression by measuring: changes in the insulin-producing cells within the pancreas, insulin resistance, and the anti-inflammatory cytokine known as adiponectin. These measurements were taken at the beginning, after three months, after six months and after nine months. Here's what they discovered: "After 9 months of treatment, 16.4 percent of subjects in the placebo group were diagnosed with T2DM, whereas none were diagnosed with T2DM in the curcumin-treated group. In addition, the curcumin-treated group showed a better overall function of β-cells, with higher HO MA -β (61.58 vs. 48.72; P < 0.01) and lower C-peptide (1.7 vs. 2.17; P < 0.05). The curcumin-treated group showed a lower level of HO MA -IR (3.22 vs. 4.04; P < 0.001) and higher adiponectin (22.46 vs. 18.45; P < 0.05) when compared with the placebo group."

Their conclusion? "A 9-month curcumin intervention in a prediabetic population significantly lowered the number of pre-diabetic individuals who eventually developed T2DM. In addition, the curcumin treatment appeared to improve overall function of β-cells, with very minor adverse effects. Therefore, this study demonstrated that the curcumin intervention in a pre-diabetic population may be beneficial."

(The full study can be seen for free on the American Diabetic Association's Diabetes Care website: http://care.diabetesjournals.org/content/35/11/2121. full online.)

This is big news since at least 40 percent of the US population between the ages of 40 and 74 is believed to be pre-diabetic, according to CDC statistics. What's even better is that turmeric powder is affordable, safe and easy to find. And, at last count, there are more than 600 potential health benefits of turmeric/curcumin, which you can read more about at the National Library of Medicine's open access database. We're covering quite a few of them in this book.

Hopefully, those who are pre-diabetic or battling full-blown diabetes will take hold of this turmeric teaching and do their bodies a favor.

What we have had tremendous results with in my office is using GHI cleanse which contains turmeric. Plus additional concentrated turmeric extract. Plus an excellent cinnamon extract product. This three pronged appraoch is great for helping to maintaining health blood glucose levels.

Plus another that works well is to use 1 ounce fresh squeezed lemon juice into 9 ounces of water sweetened with stevia.

Its great tasting lemonade that is good for you.

Resources:

[1] Somlak Chuengsamarn, Suthee Rattanamongkolgul, Rataya Luechapudiporn, Chada Phisalaphong, Siwanon Jirawatnotai. *Curcumin extract for prevention of type 2 diabetes*. Diabetes Care. 2012 Nov; 35(11):2121-7. Epub 2012 Jul 6. PMID: 22773702

[2] CDC: Dia

34 | Fructose Findings

Sugar and Cancer go Hand-in-Hand.

Hard to believe but high-fructose corn syrup is the primary source of calories in the United States , according to recent statistics, which might also explain why the prevalence of cancer in the US is on the rise. Fructose not only contains mercury, which is a known carcinogen, but also cancer cells feed on high-fructose corn syrup once it has been metabolized by the liver.

Health experts have made the connection between sugar and cancer for many years but a recent study published in the Expert Opinion on Therapeutic Targets added even more evidence that there is a definite link between excess sugar consumption and the development of cancer. Here are just some of the ways in which fructose contributes to cancer risk and other health issues, according to this recent study:

- DNA damage
- Inflammation
- Altered cellular metabolism
- Increased production of free radicals

As much as 80 percent of all cancers are "driven by either mutations or environmental factors that work to enhance or mimic the effect of insulin on the incipient tumor cells," says Lewis Cantley, director of the Cancer Center at Beth Israel Deaconnes Medical Center at Harvard Medical School. Furthermore, there have been similar findings published in Cancer Research about the way sugar is metabolized and how it actually stimulates cancer growth. But, here's something even more alarming regarding fructose. This study shows that cancer cells can easily metabolize fructose to increase reproduction. The researchers used pancreatic cancer cells in their research, which is one of the most deadly forms of cancer, and found that not only did the tumor cells feed on glucose but also the tumor cells used fructose for cell division in order to speed the growth and spread of cancer! In other words, fructose actually caused massive increase in the tumors' cell growth and overall reproduction—far beyond that of glucose.

This would be very bad news even if fructose was just mildly popular in our diets, but it has become the number one source of calories for Americans. In fact, statistics show that the average American consumes approximately 150 grams of sugar every day, which is particularly alarming when experts suggest we consume no more than 15 grams per day to avoid cancer. Even children consume large amounts of sugar daily via their juice boxes, "healthy" sports drinks, sodas and candy. Fructose is sneaky and can be in many beverage and food items that you'd never suspect, so we must be proactive about this—read labels and cut fructose from our diets once and for all. Stevia, which is a natural sweetener, is a much better choice and has zero calories. There's really no excuse for continuing to put poison into your body, so now that you know the truth about fructose, eliminate it from your life.

Sources:http://www.nytimes.com/2011/04/17/magazine/mag 17Sugar-t.html?_r=2

35 | Just Say No to GMOS

So, just what is GMO and why is it in the news so much recently? Glad you asked. A genetically modified organism (GMO) is a term that describes any food that has been genetically modified to a form that you won't find in nature. Crops are often genetically modified so they will be more hearty and resistant to viruses and insects, but studies have shown that GMOs are harmful to those who consume them, which is where the controversy began and why it continues today.

Take, for example, these groundbreaking studies:

A study recently published in *The Journal of Hematology & Thromboembolic Diseases* deals with the potential "leukemogenic" properties of the Bt toxin biopesticides engineered into most GMO food crops within the United States food supply. The study reveals that Bt may contribute to blood abnormalities ranging from anemia to hematological malignancies such as leukemia.

In addition, the researchers were finally able to disprove the prevailing myth regarding selective toxicity of Bt to insects, which is the target species of Bt. The study showed that Cry toxins were not only activated at the alkaline pH of the digestive tract of susceptible larvae, but also that Bt spore-crystals caused in vitro hemolysis in cell lines of rats, mice, sheep, horses and human erythrocytes, suggesting that the plasma membrane of susceptible cells may actually be the primary target for these toxins.

Also, this study revealed that a dose of Cry1Ab as low as 27mg/kg—the lowest tested dose—was still capable of causing hypochromic anemia in mice. (This is the same toxin that has been found in the blood of non-pregnant women, pregnant women and their fetuses in Canada , supposedly contracted through diet.)

In addition, this study totally contradicted past reports that claimed Bt toxins are generally nontoxic and rarely bio-accumulate in fatty tissue or persist in the environment after the initial exposure. This study proved that all Cry toxins tested had an even greater effect 72 hours after the initial exposure. That is exactly the opposite of what had been perpetuated in the media.

At the conclusion of this important study, the researchers said, "It is premature to consider GM toxins to be safe in mammals." Wow! Did you get that? The researchers said it may be premature to consider if GM toxins are safe for mammals; however, billions of people have already been exposed to Bt toxins! Still, despite this groundbreaking study, most biotech research scientists and industry regulators will claim GM toxins are perfectly safe. Why? Because of the well-known relationship that biotech corporations like Monsanto have with corrupt science firms who are basically paid to "prove" and "stand behind" whatever the corporations want them to prove or disprove—like the link between cancer and GMO food. The biotech companies definitely don't want that link confirmed, yet it already has been.

Just last year, the link between cancer and GMO food was established in a French study, becoming the first independent long-term animal feeding study not commissioned by the biotech corporations.

So, as you can see there are studies upon studies being done on GMOs, but only a few of them are credible because most of the faux research is being funded by the biotech industry. Some argue that we should stop waiting around for the corrupt legislative process to force manufacturers to label GMOs, and instead fight to ban GMOs once and for all before it is too late to undo the damage to our biosphere and our bodies. I'm going to let you make that call.

THE GLOBAL TIDES ARE TURNING

It seems that GMO support is waning worldwide as more and more experts are blowing the whistle on "faux research findings," causing former big buyers to back away from our GMO crops. In fact, a recent news report stated that the formerly pro-GMO Chinese government, which is one of the largest consumers of GMO food crops in the world, is beginning to crack down on GM corn shipments from the United States for not following appropriate biosafety regulations. GMWatch.org reports that China destroyed three shipments of GM corn imported from the US .

However, despite these recent drastic steps by Chinese authorities to destroy GM seeds, an article that appeared in China Daily last year revealed that the consumption of GM soybeans has become universal in China , even despite widespread public concerns that they had not been adequately safety tested. According to Shi Yan-quan, Deputy Director of Agricultural Finance and Education Dept., who was quoted in the article, over 50 million tons of GMO soybeans were imported to China in 2011 alone. The article also reveals that for eight years, 1.3 billion Chinese consumers have been consuming Monsanto's GM food crops, relying solely on biotech-funded safety evaluations, without any independent safety testing carried out by the Chinese government.

This article in China Daily was quite shocking since a 2012 study found that the Chinese print media is completely co-opted by biotech industry influence, revealing that 48.1 percent of articles were largely supportive of the GM technology research and development programs, while 51.9 percent of articles were neutral on the subject of GMOs. Sure, risks associated with GMOs were mentioned in the newspaper articles, but none of the articles took a negative tone in regards to GMOs.

So, are the tides turning? Are these recent incidents a sign that the Chinese government is beginning to take more seriously the health threats associated with the consumption of GM food? Mr. Li of the GMWatch.org believes the tides are turning. He said, "The new government's decisive move to destroy the illegal GMOs is progressive, encouraging, and satisfying," noting that it's a sign the Chinese government is keeping its promise to work for the people and the nation.

References:

- GMWatch.org , China Destroys three Shipments of GM Corn from US, May 22nd, 2013
- Translated by a Chinese citizen whose identity remains anonymous, but GMWatch refers to under the pseudonym as "Mr. Li."
- Additional important research resources on GreenMedInfo.com
  Surprise! Monsanto-Funded Research Finds Their Products Safe
  Health Guide: GMO Research
- Bélin Poletto Mezzomo, Ana Luisa Miranda-Vilela, Ingrid de Souza Freire, Lilian Carla Pereira Barbosa, Flávia Arruda Portilho. Hematotoxicity of Bacillus thuringiensis as Spore-crystal Strains Cry1Aa, Cry1Ab, Cry1Ac or Cry2Aa in Swiss Albino Mice. Journal of Hematology and Thromboembolic Diseases. 2013
- Lennart Hardell, Mikael Eriksson, Marie Nordstrom. Exposure to pesticides as risk factor for non-Hodgkin's lymphoma and hairy cell leukemia: pooled analysis of two Swedish case-control studies. Leuk Lymphoma. 2002 May;43(5):1043-9. PMID: 12148884

36 The Dangers of Weed Killers

Years ago, I told you about and warned you about the dangers of the herbicide," Round Up". Several weeks ago a story broke that revealed that Roundup, glyphosate, multiplies the growth or proliferation of breast cancer cells by a staggering 500 to 1300 %, occurring at even minuscule amounts in the parts per trillion.

The study published in the *Food and Chemical Toxicology* is titled *"Glyphosate Induces Human Breast Cancer Cells Growth Via Estrogen Receptors."*

Some additional research also links it to an increased risk of testicular cancer.

Here's the problem: With the uber- evil corporation, Monsanto, bringing us roundup- ready corn, soybeans and canola, Roundup has proliferated the eco system. It is now in our food ... in our water, and, if you are in a farming community, it is in the air! Quite frankly, this is insane!

There are so many crops that are now Round -up ready, that we are having a massive devastation to our water ways due to agricultural run- off into the streams and lakes.

In fact, due to the lies and lobbying of Monsanto, California just set limits for Roundup in the drinking water to 1,000 parts per billion; that's 1000 times higher than the amount shown to increase breast cancer growth by up to 1300%. By the way, even the EPA has set its safe limits at 700 ppb on roundup in the water.

We all know the country is in trouble. Look at all the mess going on in the media. But, why won't the media report on this study? I will tell you why again. The media is owned by the same banks that own Monsanto. I know that sounds nuts, but alternative health experts, including myself, have all but been banned on main stream media.

Years ago I appeared on what was then CBS Channel 13 in Tampa. It is now a Fox affiliate. I appeared at that time on The Kathy Fountain Show. The show received a 37% market share which was one of the highest market shares the station ever obtained.

Six months later I was asked to come back on, but I was told I could not mention Aspartame...at all...period! The owners of Aspartame, Monsanto, had told the station that it would pull all their advertising if I spoke about Aspartame again. So, I was muzzled and so was the host.

Several years later, this same station, which is now a Fox station, produced another program called "The Investigators." They did an extensive show on Bovine growth hormone. That show was also never allowed to air, due to the manufacturers of the hormone , which again, is Monsanto. Go to my website to get the direct link.

You all should know me well enough by to know that I don't make this stuff up. I don't need to make anything up. The truth is already bizarre enough.

Last year when the California consumers overwhelmingly wanted GMOS labeled and the ballot initiative failed, when the big boys like Monsanto spent tens of millions on lobbying against the initiative, it made me wonder at the time...now, I know why it failed.

Let me put it more bluntly if I can: Monsanto, GMO , Roundup and chemical assault on the USA is killing us by contributing to breast Cancer, Testicular Cancer, brain cancer...and, I am sure as we become more aware of the harmful effect it has on us, the list will probably go on and on.

Last year I wrote and showed you the tumors from mice who were fed Roundup -ready GMO corn. (I even told you that as far as I was concerned, the weeds had won. But I have concocted a new weed killer made of Vinegar and salt. It works great! A friend of mine uses diesel fuel.)

Also released a few weeks ago was another study which was done on swine being fed GMO corn. The results showed massive inflammation in the stomach and gut.

GMO feed destroys pig stomachs. They become an inflammatory mush. Photos reveal severe damage caused by GM soy and corn. This is one of the reasons so many people are having Gastrointestinal Disorders.

Friends, at the risk of sounding like a conspiracy theorist, let me tell you Margaret Sanger's Eugenics program is alive and well.

Now that I have given you the facts and the truth, please stay with me for some healthy alternatives:

1. Never eat corn, soy beans (estrogen) or canola oil or their by-products. (with the exception of vitamin E from a natural soy source)
2. Try and eat organically raised foods.
3. Take Healthmasters GHI Cleanse. Take two scoops daily for gastrointestinal inflammation.
4. Use one of our water distillers. It's simple: the ground and municipal water contain Roundup plus a lot more poison. The plastic jugs you are using from the grocery store for water probably contain BPA. If they don't contain BPA they contain plastic residue. All of this poison is terrible for your kidneys and liver.
5. Take two scoops of our organic non GMO beet crystals daily. These are great for the body.

37 | Iodine and Radiation Exposure

When the nuclear disaster happened in Japan, I told my email subscribers it was time for you to stock up Potassium Iodine. Well it's that time. At the time of that writing the reactor disaster was releasing 300,000 tons of contaminated seawater a day into the Pacific Ocean.

Therefore, I have specifically developed a Potassium Iodine product with synergistic components for maximum absorptive ability, which I have kept at an affordable price level, for the main purpose of taking for exposure to radiation.

I recommend you stock up with three bottles per family member more if you have family members who don't live with you. After The Fukushima disaster iodine prices went through the roof and supply was nonexistent. Please stock up for your family members. This is not a joke. It may save your family's life.

Here is some more technical info on the Japan disaster and the importance of getting iodine into your system as soon as possible.

As we all know the Fukushima power plant was knocked about in the huge earthquake that hit Japan. There is continued radioactive material leakage at the Fukushima Daiichi power plant..

So why would taking extra iodide protect against radiation poisoning? To answer that, we need to take a pretty big step back.

Many nuclear reactors get their energy by smacking uranium-235 with a neutron, called fission. And in a turn a single act of fission can create more than 200 million times the energy of the neutron that kicked it off in the first place. I'm not going to go into why here, but it has to do with the famous Einstein equation.

So when uranium-235 decays, it gets broken into a lot of smaller fragments. One of these is iodine-131. It's also radioactive. Out of the most common fission products of uranium, iodine is the only one that's present naturally in our bodies.

There are actually fourteen major radioactive isotopes of iodine. The majority of them are not considered dangerous, because they have very long half-lives. That's the time it takes for half the radioactive material in the element to decay.

I'm simplifying here, but you get the general idea: iodine-131 has the potential to do a lot more damage to the body, because it gives off more radiation in a short period of time.

And where it's going to do that damage is mostly in the thyroid.

That little butterfly-looking thing in your neck is the only part of the body that can absorb iodine. It pulls it out of food and, along with the amino acid tyrosine, converts it into the hormones thyroxine (T4) and triiodothyronine (T3).

T3 and T4 go off into the blood stream and the rest of the body where they oversee the conversion of oxygen and calories to energy. Every single cell in the body relies on these hormones to regulate their metabolism.

So imagine if the iodine absorbed by the body were radioactive. That is very bad and very deadly.

Iodine is pretty volatile . So if a nuclear reactor were to leak, iodine-131 might be in the air. Which people might breathe in. Which could get into their thyroids. Which could cause radiation poisoning in the short term. In the long term, breathing radioactive iodine can cause thyroid cancer, especially in kids.

To minimize the damage, people who may be/have been exposed to radiation from a power plant can take iodide pills. These work by saturating the thyroid with nice, non-radioactive iodide. That way, if any radioactive iodine does come along, the body won't absorb it — the thyroid can only absorb a finite amount of iodine at a time.

If people can get these pills 48 hours before or eight hours after radiation exposure, it can reduce thyroid uptake of iodine-131 and hopefully decrease the risk of radiation-induced thyroid cancer.

Healthmasters now carries potassium iodide. I recommend everyone keep it on hand.

38 | Study Says HPV Vaccines Do More Harm than Good

I have a friend who recently shared a story that saddened me but certainly didn't surprise me. She told how she took both of her teenage daughters to the doctor for their annual sports physicals, and by the time she had finished filling out all of the paperwork in the waiting area, her oldest daughter had already been given a Gardasil injection. When she entered the room where her daughters were being seen, she encountered her youngest daughter having a shouting match with the nurse who was insisting she also get the Gardasil injection. My friend said she calmed her daughter and told the nurse that her daughter didn't want the Gardasil injection and would not be receiving it that afternoon. To that, the nurse responded, "So you're just going to let your daughter get cervical cancer then? When you know this vaccine can keep her from such a horrible disease, why wouldn't you insist she receive it?" My friend and her youngest daughter stood their ground, but the nurse had already made her point abundantly clear. She was basically saying that anyone who doesn't force a child to get the Gardasil vaccine is a bad parent.

I'm sure this type of scenario plays out all over the country, and most parents won't stand their ground and refuse the injection, rather they succumb to the medical pressure to get the Gardasil or Cervarix vaccine for their daughters, never realizing there is strong evidence that those vaccines can produce severe and even life-threatening harm. On the flip side, there is no proof that Gardasil or Cervarix can prevent cancer any better than a decent screening program. So, why is the medical world forcing our girls to get a vaccine that is harmful and has no merit? It all comes down to this—those who are funding the studies are also the ones manufacturing the vaccines, and in the case of Gardasil, all of the authors had financial ties to the manufacturer of the Gardasil vaccine—Merck.

The ugly truth:

A report originally published in Gaia Health featured four scientists who clearly showed how science had been corrupted and misused to promote these life-altering vaccines when there is no clear evidence that Gardasil or Cervarix can prevent cancer better than a decent screening program, and definite evidence they can produce severe side effects and life-threatening harm. zIn addition, another group of scientists who had done extensive research on the topics of immunization and autoimmune disorders made the following conclusion: "Physicians should remain within the rigorous rules of evidence-based medicine, to adequately assess the risks versus the benefits of HPV vaccination." Reading through the paper, it's quite clear that they are saying the evidence does not support a positive risk-benefit ratio for the human papilloma virus (HPV) vaccines, Gardasil and Cervarix.

Their paper focuses on three young women who had normal development yet experienced ovarian failure after receiving the HPV vaccinations. All other potential causes of ovarian failure were ruled out, so they were able to conclude the vaccines had been the reason for their ovaries to fail. How many more are out there? We may never know because the way physicians treat girls who start having irregular periods is to give them hormonal drugs which ultimately mask the symptoms of ovarian failure.

There is more: The paper goes on to discuss HPV vaccines and autoimmunity.

The authors compare the three girls' symptoms to the newly-described syndrome called ASIA (Autoimmune/inflammatory syndrome induced by adjuvants), and all three fit the criteria. Included were some of those symptoms: muscle weakness, chronic fatigue, cognitive disturbances, pyrexia and more. It was determined that all three suffered from the vaccine-induced ASIA syndrome, which was difficult to identify since ASIA symptoms are often deemed irrelevant or non-vaccine related by the patients themselves or by their attending physicians. That's dangerous because those symptoms should never be ignored and are clearly associated with severely disabling conditions.

The authors point out that the literature currently documents: "... numerous cases substantiating the link between adverse immune reactions and HPV vaccines, including fatal reactions."

Citing the case of a teenage girl who suffered dizziness, prickling skin, memory lapses, excessive tiredness, night sweats, a loss of ability to use common objects, intermittent chest pain, and sudden racing heart spells after receiving the HPV vaccination, the report states that she died suddenly six months after receiving the third Gardasil vaccination. According to the documented case, the autopsy was unable to identify any toxicological, microbiological, or anatomical cause of death. However, further investigation showed that her blood and spleen had been contaminated with HPV-16 L1 gene DNA fragments, which corresponds with the fragments found in Gardasil vaccine vials from various lots.

The authors then point out that HPV vaccination has been associated with the following several autoimmune diseases: Guillain-Barré syndrome, demyelinating neuropathies, systemic lupus erythematosus, pancreatitis, vasculitis, thrombocytopenic purpura, and autoimmune hepatitis. However, the most common autoimmune disorders associated with HPV vaccines are neurological in nature.

Breaking it down, the authors reveal that several ingredients in the two HPV vaccines are known to be problematic. For example, Saccharomyces cerevisiae (common yeast), in which the Gardasil antigen is made, is known to trigger autoimmune response.

Even if that were the only problematic ingredient, that would be enough to refute the findings of a recent study that say, "there are no adverse effects whatsoever in either vaccine."

In addition, the authors of this all-important paper reveal the study is biased. Concluding the statement, "There are no adverse effects whatsoever in either vaccine" to be false. For example, only women who had been vaccinated with at least one dose were included, "thus making this particular population less sensitive for the detection of serious adverse reactions (given that such events occur with much lesser frequency when fewer doses of the vaccine are administered)." Also, the autoimmune disorders that were the primary focus of this study included rheumatological and neurological/ophthalmic; however, not a single doctor who screened the study's participants had experience in those fields. Lastly, in every clinical trial evaluating safety for both Gardasil and Cervarix, the so-called placebo groups were given injections that included an active aluminum adjuvant! Though this is a common practice in vaccine trials, it will obviously bias the results.

Can it be any wonder that these researchers have concluded that there is no evidence base to document the safety of either Gardasil or Cervarix? Clearly, any doctor who genuinely cares for patient safety must treat this lack of safety evidence as unacceptable regarding the HPV vaccines. As the authors state in their conclusion:

"Given that persistently infected women with HPV seem not to develop cancer if they are regularly screened and that the long-term clinical benefits of HPV vaccination are still a matter of speculation, a more rigorous assessment of vaccine risks and benefits is recommended. Thus, physicians should remain within the rigorous rules of evidence-based medicine, to adequately assess the risks versus the benefits of HPV vaccination."

Their final conclusion?

Indeed, the HPV vaccines appear to have failed to meet a single one of the four criteria required by the FDA for Fast Track approval.

My final conclusion is a little more direct. Why are we giving ineffective drugs to young girls that are causing them to have fertility and severe health problems including death? Is this some type of "Globalist Agenda" that has been a stated goal of the United Nations, that population controls must be put into place? Who knows? But, as you have seen throughout this book so many of the current drugs, food and water additives cause infertility.

That seems strange to me. I am not a "conspiracy theorist." I am a scientist. I look at the facts. The facts are becoming clear: It is simply that more and more women and men are becoming infertile.

Resources:

Human Papilloma Virus Vaccine and Primary Ovarian Failure: Another Facet of the Autoimmune/Inflammatory Syndrome Induced by Adjuvants; American Journal of °Reproductive Immunology; Colafrancesco S, Perricone C, Tomljenovic L, Shoenfeld Y; doi: 10.1111/aji.12151.
products of uranium-235.]

39 | Maintaining a Healthy Heart and Cardiovascular System

Not too long ago, Sharon and I were taping a television show on her cookbook, Healthy Country Cooking. What my wife and I discussed then, and have decided, is that it is easier to get folks to change their diets and, thereby, their health, by taking small steps over a longer period of time, than trying to do everything at once. One of my fellow speakers, Jim Rohn, said it so succinctly: " You can't whip a U-turn with the Queen Mary luxury cruise ship." Changes in course and directions have to be made subtlety. That is my goal for each of you. I want you and your family to realize that it doesn't have to be difficult to be healthy. Nor does it have to be miserable to be healthy. It can be fun and rewarding. But you need to make a decision. For example: If you are 20-30-40-50 pounds overweight and you feel terrible, how bad does it have to get before you decide to make different choices? Remember the choices you have made have given you your current results. One definition of insanity is to expect different results from the same action. Always remember we are literally what we eat! Our bodies do their best to break down and absorb nutrients from the food we eat to build healthy cells. The problem is that much of our food has no nutritional value. Our bodies simply cannot make healthy cells. We literally live and die at the cellular level ,and many of our cells become sick and die from the lack of nutrients.

Maintaining a healthy heart:

If you want to avoid a stroke, heart attack or dying from Americas #1 killer, you probably need to forget all the mainstream information you have heard. The truth of the matter is very eye- opening. Heart disease was basically unheard of in 1910, only causing about 3000 deaths annually in the United States. Then, by 1930, statistics jumped to 500.000 deaths. By 1960 and despite spending hundreds of billions, if not trillions of dollars since then, it has never decreased below that level. Several years ago the rates hit one million per year, which is one every 33 seconds. Many of us have realized something is wrong, very wrong.

First, let me tell you why there was such a huge spike from 1930 - 1960. That was the era junk food (processed) production went crazy in this country. That is also the era that Hydrogenated oils were first used. Hydrogenated oils were first used as a substitute for butter. During the war there was a scarcity of butter. What scientists discovered was if they took corn oil and heated it, then bubbled hydrogen through it using nickel as a catalyst, they could take the liquid corn oil and turn it into a solid fat (Crisco). Then yellow food coloring could be added producing a butter substitute, (margarine). The problem is this type of fat is not found in nature. It is called a trans fat and is extremely toxic. It causes heart disease, cancer and infertility just for starters. Finally, this year the USDA has required all manufacturers to list the amount of trans fat in their products. However, some of the manufactures have already found ways to hide this on their labels.

So here's the fact: The processed foods that we are eating are causing almost all of the deaths from cardiovascular diseases. Notice I have not mentioned cholesterol, tryglycerides or blood pressure. That's right, because these three can be controlled through dietary changes. By the way, half the people who die of heart attacks have normal blood pressure, cholesterol and triglycerides. Many of them, just prior to dropping dead, have had physicals, EKG's and stress tests showing that their hearts were in great shape. Interestingly, the major drug companies do not want you to have these statistics. I wrote in my book, Maximum Energy (which by the way, is an international best seller covering in detail the top ten foods never to eat) about a coach I had in high school. His name was Tom. He was a great guy. One day I was speaking to him in the local gym telling him how good he looked. His comment was, " I'm 62 years old. The doctor told me I have the body of a 42 year old." He was curling 150 pounds for 10 reps. He was amazing. Three days later, he was dead. He had a massive heart attack. The entire community was devastated.

While the medical community, in confusion, has known about unprecedented, heart attack rates for years, they literally have not known why. Well, I've got good news for you! A new study out of Paris is shedding light on people, primarily men, who are dropping dead from heart attacks for no apparent reason.

It seems from the Paris study that one, if not the primary problems, is that these victims have high levels of Non-esterified fatty acids (NEFA) in their blood. It can cause dangerous ventricular dysrhythmias if you have coronary artery disease and low oxygen delivery to your heart. STOP!

Don't start fussing, as I know what you are thinking: " He is doing it again. I don't want this technical stuff. I'm not a biochemist." Okay, you are so right. I'll make it easy. By the way, just for the old university memories, I do enjoy talking and writing like that. But I have a confession to make. My wife always fusses at me when I do. So here's the bottom line: High levels of NEFA's are caused by too much Omega 6 in the diet. Omega 6 comes from corn, safflower, sunflower and canola oils.

My recommendations for a healthy heart:

1. Start taking the **Cod Blue Ice** every day. By taking one teaspoon once or twice a day, it literally improves vascular integrity and provides anti-inflammatory effects. Remember cardio-vascular disease has been linked to inflammation. One of the bio markers that are used to identify early warning signs of potential cardiovascular disease is called CRP (C-Reactive Protein). This inflammatory marker indicates potential cardio-vascular disease. Notice that I really haven't talked much about cholesterol. Here's why: Cholesterol is an anti-inflammatory product that reduces inflammation. The body produces cholesterol as a defense mechanism to reduce inflammation. So, what does mainstream medicine do?

It gives us statin drugs to reduce our cholesterol. These statin drugs cause muscle wasting (Myopathy). which makes the heart disease much worse, plus they cause cancer. Fish oil lowers CRP naturally, which then gets the body to reduce cholesterol to a normal level.

It really is that simple. Now if you are taking prescription drugs. Don't stop on your own, but go to your doctor to have him help you reduce or eliminate your dosage. If he won't help, find a medical doctor who will. If you are still worried about cholesterol, there are two products, which work great without causing myopathy.

2. **Body Balance HEMMLA**: This helps maintain healthy cholesterol. Healthmasters HEMMLA is an omega-3 Phospholipid concentrate. Super Critical-Solvent Free Extraction. It contains the Highest Yield of Phospholipid, EPA/DHA and Astaxanthin. Healthmasters HEMMLA is the First Medical Food Sourced from Krill.

3. **Cholesterol-X**: It is policosanol and a patented magnesium chelate. This acts to maintain healthy cholesterol without causing side effects. It helps to reduce the liver's production of cholesterol.

4. **Super Potent E**: This is a mixed tocopheral product, which is high in gamma E. This is the most potent E to protect against LDL cholesterol (the bad one) breakdown. When you oxidize or breakdown the LDL cholesterol,l it's like turning little razor blades loose in your arteries.

This oxidized LDL cholesterol actually creates lesions (little cuts) in the blood vessels. These little cuts then form scars, which can cause blockages in the arteries, heart disease and heart attacks. I recommend 1600 iu for men and 800 iu for women daily. I have been taking 1600 iu for 25 years. The study several years ago saying Vitamin E was bad used chemically produced cheap synthetic E. No study has ever shown that natural mixed tocopheral E does anything but good. The cost is $19.00 for 60 capsules.

5. **Magnesium and Malate Acid**: These are natural muscle relaxants, which help to lower blood pressure. It also uses patented Albion chelate minerals, which are absorbed by the body as food. Remember metallic minerals are rock and are absorbed very poorly by the body. I go into detail on the different types of minerals in my home study series "Forever Fit at 20 -30 -40 -50 and beyond." Magnesium also helps to lower blood pressure and allows more oxygen to be delivered to the heart. If you are taking Cholesterol-X, you will not need this. The cost is$26.95 for 120 capsules.

6. Use foods high in Omega 3 such as fresh wild Salmon (never use farm raised Salmon). Also, good plant sources are leaf lettuce, Flax seeds and Walnuts. Plus, remember to use Olive oil, Grape seed oil, Coconut oil or organic butter in your cooking . It's important to get as much Omega 3 as possible.

40 | Could Calcium Kill?

You think you're doing a good thing for your body by faithfully taking your calcium supplement every day, but as it turns out, you could be setting yourself up for a heart attack. Recent research published in Heart shared the findings of two controversial studies regarding calcium supplementation and heart attack risk, originally made public in the British Medical Journal in 2012. Researchers found a 24 to 27 percent increase of heart attack for people taking 500 mg of elemental calcium daily. And that's not all. A newer study involving 24,000 people between the ages of 35 and 64 revealed that those who took a regular calcium supplement were 86 percent more likely to have a heart attack than those who didn't take any calcium supplements.

These findings really shouldn't come as such a big surprise since we have long administered coronary and cardiac calcium scans in order to determine a person's risk of future cardiovascular events and/or cardiac mortality. The bottom line is this: Calcium of the wrong kind in the wrong place often results in negative health events. In fact, many experts in the field of nutrition have long been discouraging the use of elemental calcium supplementation, which is calcium from limestone, oyster shells, egg shells and bone meal (hydroxyl apatite). And, you really don't have to be "an expert" to figure out that consuming rocks and shells is probably not such a great idea. So, why do we do it?

Part of the popularity of taking elemental calcium supplements stems from the excessive promotional efforts of conventional health organizations like the National Osteoporosis Foundation. But guess who sponsors that foundation? Oscal and Citrical, which are two major calcium manufacturers. Also fueling the fire of the elemental calcium supplements craze is the World Health Organization. Back in 1994, the World Health Organization drastically changed the new definition of "normal" bone density for women by using a 25-year-old woman's bone density as the new standard for all women, no matter their age. This was a game changer since a 25-year-old woman is at peak bone mass in her life cycle at that particular age. Thus, the normal, gradual loss of bone mineral density that comes with aging was now seen as a disease that required treatment when in reality, it was just the normal aging process. Suddenly, millions of women felt forced into taking unnecessary and potentially dangerous "bone-building" drugs and elemental calcium supplements to increase their bone mineral density because they now had been "diagnosed" with osteopenia or osteoporosis even though their bone density was truly normal for their age, gender and ethnicity.

Fast forward from that 1994 decision: Figuring in the almost 20 years of force-feeding women bone-building drugs and elemental calcium supplements, and today we have women who are dying prematurely from calcium-induced heart attacks and/or high bone mineral density associated malignant breast cancer—the number one and number two killers of women today. So, I ask you this: Would it be better to risk fracturing a bone due to low bone mineral density or risk dying from a calcium-induced heart attack? That's a no-brainer, isn't it?

Furthermore, even if you don't suffer from a calcium-induced heart attack or succumb to bone mineral density associated malignant breast cancer, you are setting yourself up for many other health problems because when inorganic, elemental calcium travels to the wrong place or in excessive amounts, bad things happen.

Understand that elemental calcium is not bound to amino acids, lipids or glyconutrients found in food because we aren't getting it from food; we're getting it from shells and rocks. Without the proper delivery system, the calcium can end up in excessive amounts in various parts of the body such as the bowel or the kidneys causing constipation and kidney stones. Or, even worse, high levels of calcium can settle in the blood and cause blood clots, hypertension, arrhythmias or a coronary artery spasm. Also, the breasts are especially sensitive to excessive amounts of calcium known as ectopic calcification.

This may explain why women with the highest bone density (often obtained through massive, lifelong calcium supplementation) have up to 300 percent higher incidence of malignant breast cancer. Too much elemental calcium might also be to blame for an increasingly strange phenomenon called "brain gravel," in which autopsied patients have been found to have pebble-size calcium deposits throughout their brains.

We have become a calcium-fixated culture, taking mega doses of elemental calcium, all the while thinking we're doing a good thing for our bodies. We now have proof that we're not, so stop taking it! Stay away from inorganic calcium supplements and instead ingest your calcium from legumes and leafy greens. If you are a woman, I suggest if you are going to take calcium supplements that you only use products such as our Healthmasters Bone Support. This is what my wife Sharon uses. This product is chelated so that it is absorbed properly. The studies referred to above used calcium from "rock" sources. These types of rock products which are found in major health food stores and discount chains are dangerous and ineffective. Men by the way, should never take any calcium supplements. (Unless they are trying to maintain their pH levels and then only temporarily. Plus there are better ways for men and women to balance pH levels.) Men simply do not need them. Obtaining calcium needs for men can be easily obtained through food sources. Let me put it to you more directly: Men if you take calcium supplements, you will massively increase your risk of heart attack. Do not do it! If you are concerned about calcium, you need to find a source of organic grass- fed non- homogenized milk and drink a glass occasionally. By the way, that is also great for women. That's what I do. Our children drink this milk daily.

One final comment on this topic: For years I have promoted the use of Healthmasters distilled water. This is one of the primary reasons why I believe so strongly about distilled water. Regular well and municipal water contains all types of poison including elemental calcium. In other words the water contains dissolved rock. When you drink it, as this article clearly proves, it can end up in the soft tissue. Have you ever seen a hot water heater core that is completely blocked by what looks like layers upon layers of calcium or rock? This is what can happen to your arteries. That is why it is called " hardening of the arteries." Your arteries get lined with rock until a blockage occurs. It really is that simple. I have been drinking Healthmasters distilled water for 30 years. I feel great. My mental acuity is still through the roof. If any of you have seen my latest TV broadcast made at the age of 57, you will attest to that. Remember, one of the primary causes of senile dementia is a reduced blood flow to the brain. Layers of calcium reduce blood flow. This reduced blood flow reduces oxygen flow to the brain. Combined with aluminum and fluoride (both neuro toxins are removed by distillation) in the water which lowers IQ scores. It is no wonder people in their 20's are being diagnosed with mental disorders which were once reserved for the elderly.

Resources:

• BMJ 2010; 341 doi: 10.1136/bmj.c3691 (Published 29 July 2010)
• Calcium supplements with or without vitamin D and risk of cardiovascular events: reanalysis of the Women's Health Initiative limited access dataset and meta-analysis. BMJ. 2011;342:d2040. Epub 2011 Apr 19. PMID: 2150521

41 | Alzheimer's Solutions Might Be in Your Spice Cabinet

Alzheimer's Disease (AD), which is the most common form of dementia, is on the rise at an alarming rate. Chances are, you may know someone that suffers from AD. It's so common anymore, that it's almost considered a part of growing old, and that shouldn't be the case. A 2006 study reported that 26 million people throughout the world had AD at that time and predicted that by 2050, that statistic would triple. If that happens, roughly one in every 85 people will suffer from AD.

Because AD is increasing in numbers in the so-called developed countries of the world, interest in doing something about it has also increased. The search is on for safe and effective preventative and therapeutic interventions. Experts are searching for answers to this health crisis within both the conventional medical field, as well as turning to alternative options.

At this point; however, conventional drug-based treatments haven't been very effective because the medications being used to treat the symptoms often cause seizures in patients, according to World Health Organization post-marketing surveillance statistics. So, many are opting for safe, natural and effective therapies to help alleviate the symptoms of AD. Surprisingly, one of the most effective natural treatments can be found in your spice cabinet: The miracle spice, Turmeric.

Recently, a study was published in the journal Ayu titled, "Effects of turmeric (GHI cleanse) on Alzheimer's disease with behavioral and psychological symptoms of dementia," that featured three AD treatments can be found in your spice cabinet: The miracle spice, Turmeric.patients whose behavioral symptoms were improved remarkably as a result of taking 764 milligrams of turmeric for 12 weeks. Quoting the study, it said: "All three patients exhibited irritability, agitation, anxiety and apathy; two patients suffer from urinary incontinence and wonderings. They were prescribed turmeric powder capsules and started recovering from these symptoms without any adverse reaction in the clinical symptom and laboratory data."

The findings went on to say that after only three months of treatment, the patients' symptoms and the burden on their caregivers were drastically decreased. And, after taking turmeric for more than a year, all three were able to recognize their families. Obviously, this natural approach of dealing with AD has proven highly effective—both in treating and preventing the dreaded disease. For example, turmeric contains compounds such as curcumin, tetrahydrocurcumin, demethoxycurcumin and bisdemethoxycurcumin which attack the root of AD by preventing the formation of β-amyloid protein.

Also, curcuminoids are able to save long-term potentiation (functional memory) damaged by amyloid peptide, as well as reverse physiological damage by restoring neuritis and disrupting existing plaques. In addition, curcumin is known for its higher binding affinity for iron and copper over zinc, which may offer protection in regards to AD since iron-mediated damage is thought to play a pathological role.

More Super Spices:

Current research reveals there may be as many as 97 natural substances that could help in the battle against AD, with turmeric (curcumin) leading the pack. Here are a few natural AD fighters with proven track records.

- **Coconut Oil:** This oil has helped improve symptoms of cognitive decline by increasing brain-boosting ketone bodies. And it works fast, too, with only one dose and within only two hours.
- **Cocoa:** A 2009 study discovered that cocoa procyanidins may actually protect against lipid peroxidation that is related to neuronal cell death in AD.
- **Sage**: According to a 2003 study, sage extract has therapeutic merit for patients with mild to moderate AD.
- **Folic acid**: Most of the positive research on this B vitamin has been on the semi-synthetic version that sometimes has adverse side effects; however, if you get your Vitamin B from green leafy vegetables, the B vitamins (Folic acid, B6 and B12) will have more value in preventing and treating AD.
- **Resveratrol**: Found mostly in grapes, wine, peanuts and chocolate, this compound has several anti-AD properties.
- **Gingko biloba:** is one of the few herbs proven to be equally as effective as the pharmaceutical drug Aricept in treating and improving symptoms of AD.
- **Melissa offinalis**: Also known as Lemon Balm, this herb has been found helpful therapeutically for patients with mild to moderate AD.
- **Saffron:** This herb is very comparable to the drug donepezil in the treatment of mild-to-moderate Alzheimer's disease.

Of course, if you or someone you love is currently taking prescribed medication for AD, don't go off of the medication cold turkey without first consulting with a doctor. Also, remember that incorporating turmeric and some of these other spices and vitamins into your daily diet is a good idea because you can ward off many diseases and more than likely NOT be that one person in 85 who is diagnosed with AD. In other words, mine your goldmine—spice cabinet—before taking other drastic measures. Your body will thank you.

One final note concerning this topic: I am going to tell you this over and over again until hopefully it clicks. Aluminum and fluoride have to be avoided. These are both neuro toxins.

In addition thiomersal, also known as mercury has to be avoided. It is also a deadly neuro toxin. If you are getting a yearly flu shot chances are you are injecting mercury into your body. The multi- vile flu shot uses mercury as a sterilant. Plus, it contains an adjuvant which can cause brain inflammation. I do not do any shots unless I personally check the vile for mercury.

The only shots that I would do would be a clean (free of mercury) tetanus shot or antibiotics. By the way I have done neither in many years. I keep my immune system strong with vitamins C, D3 and probiotics.

Resources:

• Ron Brookmeyer, Elizabeth Johnson, Kathryn Ziegler-Graham, H Michael Arrighi. Forecasting the global burden of Alzheimer's disease. Alzheimers Dement. 2007 Jul ;3(3):186-91. PMID: 19595937
• Nozomi Hishikawa, Yoriko Takahashi, Yoshinobu Amakusa, Yuhei Tanno, Yoshitake Tuji, Hisayoshi Niwa, Nobuyuki Murakami, U K Krishna. Effects of turmeric on Alzheimer's disease with behavioral and psychological symptoms of dementia. Ayu. 2012 Oct ;33(4):499-504. PMID: 23723666
• V Chandra, R Pandav, H H Dodge, J M Johnston, S H Belle, S T DeKosky, M Ganguli. Incidence of Alzheimer's disease in a rural community in India: the Indo-US study. Neurology. 2001 Sep 25 ;57(6):985-9. PMID: 11571321
• GreenMedInfo.com, Declaring Chemical Warfare Against Alzheimer's.
• GreenMedInfo.com, Turmeric's Neuroprotective Properties (114 study abstracts)
• Laura Zhang, Milan Fiala, John Cashman, James Sayre, Araceli Espinosa, Michelle Mahanian, Justin Zaghi, Vladimir Badmaev, Michael C Graves, George Bernard, Mark Rosenthal. Curcuminoids enhance amyloid-beta uptake by macrophages of Alzheimer's disease patients. J Alzheimers Dis. 2006 Sep;10(1):1-7. PMID: 16988474
• Ava Masoumi, Ben Goldenson, Senait Ghirmai, Hripsime Avagyan, Justin Zaghi, Ken Abel, Xueying Zheng, Araceli Espinosa-Jeffrey, Michelle Mahanian, Phillip T Liu, Martin Hewison, Matthew Mizwickie, John Cashman, Milan Fiala. 1alpha,25-dihydroxyvitamin D3 interacts with curcuminoids to stimulate amyloid-beta clearance by macrophages of Alzheimer's disease patients. J Alzheimers Dis. 2009 Jul;17(3):703-17. PMID: 19433889
• Hongying Liu, Zhong Li, Donghai Qiu, Qiong Gu, Qingfeng Lei, Li Mao. The inhibitory effects of different curcuminoids onβ-amyloid protein, β-amyloid precursor protein and β-site amyloid precursor protein cleaving enzyme 1 in swAPP HEK293 cells. Int Dent J. 1996 Feb;46(1):22-34. PMID: 20727383

- Shilpa Mishra, Mamata Mishra, Pankaj Seth, Shiv Kumar Sharma. Tetrahydrocurcumin confers protection against amyloidβ-induced toxicity. Neuroreport. 2010 Nov 24. Epub 2010 Nov 24. PMID: 21116204

- Xiao-Yan Qin, Yong Cheng, Long-Chuan Yu. Potential protection of curcumin against intracellular amyloid beta-induced toxicity in cultured rat prefrontal cortical neurons. Neurosci Lett. 2010 Aug 9;480(1):21-4. PMID: 20638958

- Hong-Mei Wang, Yan-Xin Zhao, Shi Zhang, Gui-Dong Liu, Wen-Yan Kang, Hui-Dong Tang, Jian-Qing Ding, Sheng-Di Chen. PPARgamma agonist curcumin reduces the amyloid-beta-stimulated inflammatory responses in primary astrocytes. J Alzheimers Dis. 2010;20(4):1189-99. PMID: 20413894

- G P Lim, T Chu , F Yang, W Beech, S A Frautschy, G M Cole. The curry spice curcumin reduces oxidative damage and amyloid pathology in an Alzheimer transgenic mouse. J Neurosci. 2001 Nov 1;21(21):8370-7. PMID: 11606625

- Xiao-Yan Qin, Yong Cheng, Long-Chuan Yu. Potential protection of curcumin against intracellular amyloid beta-induced toxicity in cultured rat prefrontal cortical neurons. Neurosci Lett. 2010 Aug 9;480(1):21-4. PMID: 20638958

- D S Kim, S Y Park, J K Kim. Curcuminoids from Curcuma longa L. (Zingiberaceae) that protect PC12 rat pheochromocytoma and normal human umbilical vein endothelial cells from betaA(1-42) insult. Neurosci Lett. 2001 Apr 27;303(1):57-61. PMID: 11297823

- R Douglas Shytle, Paula C Bickford, Kavon Rezai-zadeh, L Hou, Jin Zeng, Jun Tan, Paul R Sanberg, Cyndy D Sanberg, Bill Roschek, Ryan C Fink, Randall S Alberte. Optimized turmeric extracts have potent anti-amyloidogenic effects. Curr Alzheimer Res. 2009 Dec;6(6):564-71. PMID: 19715544

- Fusheng Yang, Giselle P Lim, Aynun N Begum, Oliver J Ubeda, Mychica R Simmons, Surendra S Ambegaokar, Pingping P Chen, Rakez Kayed, Charles G Glabe, Sally A Frautschy, Gregory M Cole. Curcumin inhibits formation of amyloid beta oligomers and fibrils, binds plaques, and reduces amyloid in vivo. Neurochem Int. 2009 Mar-Apr;54(3-4):199-204. Epub 2008 Nov 30. PMID: 15590663

- Can Zhang, Andrew Browne, Daniel Child, Rudolph E Tanzi. Curcumin decreases amyloid-beta peptide levels by attenuating the maturation of amyloid-beta precursor protein. Gastroenterology. 2006 Jan;130(1):120-6. PMID: 20622013

- Ranjit K Giri, Vikram Rajagopal, Vijay K Kalra. Curcumin, the active constituent of turmeric, inhibits amyloid peptide-induced cytochemokine gene expression and CCR5-mediated chemotaxis of THP-1 monocytes by modulating early growth response-1 transcription factor. J Neurochem. 2004 Dec;91(5):1199-210. PMID: 15569263

- Touqeer Ahmed, Anwarul-Hassan Gilani, Narges Hosseinmardi, Saeed Semnanian, Syed Ather Enam, Yaghoub Fathollahi. Curcuminoids rescue long-term potentiation impaired by amyloid peptide in rat hippocampal slices. Synapse. 2010 Oct 20. Epub 2010 Oct 20. PMID: 20963814

- M Garcia-Alloza, L A Borrelli, A Rozkalne, B T Hyman, B J Bacskai. Curcumin labels amyloid pathology in vivo, disrupts existing plaques, and partially restores distorted neurites in an Alzheimer mouse model. J Neurochem. 2007 Aug;102(4):1095-104. Epub 2007 Apr 30. PMID: 17472706

- Larry Baum, Alex Ng. Curcumin interaction with copper and iron suggests one possible mechanism of action in Alzheimer's disease animal models. J Alzheimers Dis. 2004 Aug;6(4):367-77; discussion 443-9. PMID: 15345806

- Silvia Mandel, Tamar Amit, Orit Bar-Am, Moussa B H Youdim. Iron dysregulation in Alzheimer's disease: multimodal brain permeable iron chelating drugs, possessing neuroprotective-neurorescue and amyloid precursor protein-processing regulatory activities as therapeutic agents. Prog Neurobiol. 2007 Aug;82(6):348-60. Epub 2007 Jun 19. PMID: 17659826

- Mark A Reger, Samuel T Henderson, Cathy Hale, Brenna Cholerton, Laura D Baker, G S Watson, Karen Hyde, Darla Chapman, Suzanne Craft. Effects of beta-hydroxybutyrate on cognition in memory-impaired adults. Neurobiol Aging. 2004 Mar;25(3):311-4. PMID: 15123336
- Eun Sun Cho, Young Jin Jang, Nam Joo Kang, Mun Kyung Hwang, Yong Taek Kim, Ki Won Lee, Hyong Joo Lee. Cocoa procyanidins attenuate 4-hydroxynonenal-induced apoptosis of PC12 cells by directly inhibiting mitogen-activated protein kinase kinase 4 activity. Free Radic Biol Med. 2009 May 15;46(10):1319-27. Epub 2009 Feb 25. PMID: 19248828
- S Akhondzadeh, M Noroozian, M Mohammadi, S Ohadinia , A H Jamshidi, M Khani. Salvia officinalis extract in the treatment of patients with mild to moderate Alzheimer's disease: a double blind, randomized and placebo-controlled trial. J Clin Pharm Ther. 2003 Feb;28(1):53-9. PMID: 12605619
- Celeste A de Jager, Abderrahim Oulhaj, Robin Jacoby, Helga Refsum, A David Smith. Cognitive and clinical outcomes of homocysteine-lowering B-vitamin treatment in mild cognitive impairment: a randomized controlled trial. Int J Geriatr Psychiatry. 2011 Jul 21. Epub 2011 Jul 21. PMID: 21780182
- GreenMedInfo.com, Resveratrol's Anti-Alzheimer's properties
- S Yancheva, R Ihl, G Nikolova, P Panayotov, S Schlaefke , R Hoerr,. Ginkgo biloba extract EGb 761(R), donepezil or both combined in the treatment of Alzheimer's disease with neuropsychiatric features: a randomised, double-blind, exploratory trial. Aging Ment Health. 2009 Mar;13(2):183-90. PMID: 19347685
- M Mazza, A Capuano, P Bria, S Mazza . Ginkgo biloba and donepezil: a comparison in the treatment of Alzheimer's dementia in a randomized placebo-controlled double-blind study. Eur J Neurol. 2006 Sep;13(9):981-5. PMID: 16930364
- S Akhondzadeh, M Noroozian, M Mohammadi, S Ohadinia , A H Jamshidi, M Khani. Melissa officinalis extract in the treatment of patients with mild to moderate Alzheimer's disease: a double blind, randomized, placebo controlled trial. J Neurol Neurosurg Psychiatry. 2003

42 | Children's Vitamins: Make Wise Decisions Concerning Children

"We are Flintstones™ kids — 10 million strong and growing." You're singing that little commercial jingle in your head right now, aren't you? The Flintstones Children's Vitamins have been around quite a long time, and they are marketed very well. It is no wonder they are the number one children's vitamin brand in the United States. However, just because you can sing the well-known jingle does not make them healthy for the children in your life. Actually, this ever popular brand of children's vitamins features several unhealthy ingredients.

That may be shocking news to you because Bayer, the global pharmaceutical company that makes Flintstones Vitamins™, makes this proud declaration about their vitamins: "Pediatricians' number one choice!" And, you would think that pediatricians would only back a children's vitamin that was good for their patients, right? Well, I'll let the facts speak for themselves and you can draw your own conclusion on that one.

Flintstones Vitamins™, as yummy as they may taste, are filled with harmful ingredients such as the following: Aspartame, Cupric Oxide, artificial coloring agents, Zinc Oxide, Sorbitol, Ferrous Fumarate, Hydrogenated oil and GMO corn starch. Let's take a closer look at each of these ingredients and see if they are chemicals you wish to be putting into your children.

- **Aspartame**: A synthetic combination of the amino acids aspartic acid and 1-phenylalanine , and aspartame is known to convert into highly toxic methanol and formaldehyde once it's inside the human body. Furthermore, aspartame has been connected to more than forty horrible health effects, including neurotoxicity and carcinogenicity. [1.] Why would anyone put this harmful chemical into a children's vitamin — especially when there are healthier alternatives? Why not use non-toxic, non-synthetic sweeteners like stevia?

- **Cupric Oxide**: Each serving of Flintstones Complete Chewable Vitamins contains 2mg of Cupric Oxide, which is a very detrimental mineral. In fact, it has been used as a pigment in ceramics and in the manufacturing of rayon fabric and dry cell batteries, so why would we ever want to ingest it? So, it's quite understandable why the European Union's " Dangerous Substance Directive," which is one of the main EU laws concerning chemical safety, lists Cupric Oxide as a hazardous substance. The European Union classifies it as both "harmful", and "dangerous for the environment."
- **Coal Tar Artificial Coloring Agents**: You may already know this since hyperactivity disorder in children has been in the news a lot lately, but synthetic dyes have been proven to cause Attention Deficit Hyperactivity Disorder (ADHD). It gets worse. Studies have also shown that the neurotoxicity of artificial food coloring agents increases when mixed with aspartame, thereby, making it a double whammy.
- **Zinc Oxide**: Just the mention of Zinc Oxide probably conjures up a memory of your mom rubbing a white, smelly paste substance all over your nose and forehead so you wouldn't get sunburned. Well, each serving of Flintstones Complete Chewable Vitamins is made up of 12 mg of Zinc Oxide. What is more puzzling is this: The EU's Dangerous Substance Directive classifies it as an environmental hazard and dangerous for the environment. So, how can Zinc Oxide be dangerous for the environment, but totally fine if our children ingest it? It can't! It's much better to ingest supplemental Zinc, especially the organically-bound kind called chelated, which is connected to an amino acid like Glycine. It is much less toxic and more biodegradable.
- **Sorbitol**: A synthetic sugar substitute which is classified as a sugar alcohol. Sorbitol has been linked to gastrointestinal problems as slight as abdominal pain to the more serious irritable bowel syndrome. It's questionable whether sorbitol should be consumed by anyone, much less children.
- **Ferrous Fumarate**: If you visit the Flintstones Vitamins' website, there is a warning posted about this particular chemical, stating that while it's impossible to die from consuming iron from food, Ferrous Fumarate is an industrial mineral that is not found in nature as a food product. In fact, Ferrous Fumarate is so toxic that accidental overdoses of products containing this chemical are a leading cause of fatal poisoning in children younger than six. The manufacturer goes on to warn, "Keep this product out of reach of children. In case of accidental over dose, call a doctor or poison control center immediately."
- **Hydrogenated Soybean Oil**: It's hard to believe that anything containing Hydrogenated Oil would be marketed to children, and I find it highly offensive. Did you know that hydrogenated soybean oil has been linked to more than twelve serious health issues from coronary artery disease to

fatty liver disease to cancer? Consumption of these semi-synthetic fatty acids has also been associated with violent behavior. So the big question is, "Why are we putting them in children's vitamins?"

- **GMO Corn Starch**: Backers of these popular vitamins would argue that the small amount of GMO corn starch in this product is too slight to be an issue, but I disagree. It's a matter of being honest with consumers—us—and revealing the whole truth when labeling their products. For example, the "Vitamin C" which is listed as Ascorbic Acid is most likely produced from GMO corn. Only by knowing the background story are you able to really understand these sneaky labeling issues: Bayer's Agbiotech division, Bayer CropScience, spent $381,600 to defeat the Proposition 37, GMO labeling bill in California. Interesting, isn't it? I believe that parents have the right to know the truth, so they can make wise decisions for their children. They have the right to know the dangers of genetically modified foods and the agrichemicals that contaminate them. Let's be real! GMO corn starch is GMO, period. The Flintstones Vitamins need to reflect that truth in their labeling.

The Bayer Health Science's Flintstones Vitamins product page is quite convincing, making parents and healthcare providers feel all warm and fuzzy inside, but it's very misleading when you really know the facts. The text reads, "82% of kids aren't eating all of their veggies. Without enough vegetables, kids may not be getting all of the nutrients they need," which implies that by taking their Flintstones Vitamins, that will somehow bridge the nutritional gap. This is not true, so do not fall for their misleading marketing copy. Make wise decisions—especially where your children are concerned.

Resources:

- GreenMedInfo.com, " Adverse Health Effects of Aspartame."
- FlinstonesVitamins.com, " FLINSTONES Complete Chewable Vitamin , Nutritional Info Overview."
- Karen Lau, W Graham McLean, Dominic P Williams, C Vyvyan Howard. " Synergistic interactions between commonly used food additives in a developmental neurotoxicity test." Toxicol Sci. 2006 Mar, 90(1):178-87. Epub, 2005 Dec 13. PMID: 16352620
- GreenMedInfo.com ," Sorbitol's Adverse Health Effects."
- GreenMedInfo.com , " Health Effects of Hydrogenated Oil."
- Lorson, BA, Melgar-Quinonez, HR, Taylor CA. "Correlates of fruit and vegetable intakes in US children. The Journal of American Diet Association. 2009; 109(3):474-478. Jul;74(7):863-6. PMID: 12810768
- Shahin Akhondzadeh, Mehdi Shafiee Sabet, Mohammad Hossein Harirchian, Mansoreh Togha, Hamed Cheraghmakani, Soodeh Razeghi, Seyyed Shamssedin Hejazi, Mohammad Hossein Yousefi, Roozbeh Alimardani, Amirhossein Jamshidi, Shams-Ali Rezazadeh, Aboulghasem Yousefi, Farhad Zare, Atbin Moradi, Ardalan Vossoughi. A 22-week, multicenter, randomized, double-blind controlled trial of Crocus sativus in the treatment of mild-to-moderate Alzheimer's disease. Psychopharmacology (Berl). 2010 Jan;207(4):637-43. Epub 200

43 Turmeric: The Plant that Packs a Powerful Punch against Disease

If you could take a natural supplement instead of a prescribed medication, and it was proven to give better treatment results without the harmful side effects of the prescribed drug, wouldn't you do it? Of course you would, and so would I. That's why turmeric is gaining so much attention today. In fact, because of its healing properties, turmeric has become one of the most researched plants in existence (animal studies). Its medicinal properties—primarily curcumin—have been the topic of more than 5,600 peer-reviewed, published biomedical studies. Did you know a five-year long research of turmeric has pinpointed more than 600 potential preventative and therapeutic usages of this natural nutritional supplement. It's true! Not only that, turmeric has 175 positive physiological effects.

Studies have shown that this very special spice favorably compares to many commonly prescribed drugs, but without the negative effects of the drugs. We're going to explore some of those in this chapter:

- **Lipitor/Atorvastatin (cholesterol medication)**: According to a 2008 study published in the journal Drugs in R & D, a standardized preparation of curcuminoids from Turmeric performed much like Lipitor on endothelial dysfunction, which is the underlying pathology of blood vessels that results in atherosclerosis as it pertains to reductions in inflammation and oxidative stress in Type 2 diabetic sufferers. [i]
- **Corticosteroids (steroid medications)**: A 1999 study published in The Journal of Phytotherapy Research discovered that the primary polyphenol in turmeric, the saffron colored pigment known as curcumin, worked effectively like steroids in the management of chronic anterior uveitis, an inflammatory eye disease.[ii] Furthermore, a 2008 study published

in Critical Care Medicine found that curcumin compared favorably to the corticosteroid drug dexamethasone when tested in animals as an alternative therapy for preserving lung transplantation-associated injury by down-regulating inflammatory genes.[iii] Also, a 2003 study published in Cancer Letters found that curcumin also worked well—much like dexamethasone—in a lung ischaemia-repurfusion injury model.[iv]

- **Prozac/Fluoxetine & Imipramine (antidepressants)**: According to a 2011 study published in Acta Poloniae Pharmaceutica, curcumin proved beneficial as a substitute for both drugs in reducing depressive behavior in the animals that were tested.[v]
- **Aspirin (blood thinner)**: According to a 1986 in- vitro and ex- vivo study published in Arzneimittelforschung, researchers discovered that curcumin has anti-platelet and prostacyclin modulating effects, indicating it may have value for patients prone to vascular thrombosis and those requiring anti-arthritis therapy.[vi]
- **Non-steroidal anti-inflammatory drugs (NSAIDs)**: Millions take NSAIDs daily for arthritis and related inflammatory conditions, completely unaware that safer natural alternatives such as curcumin are readily available and very effective.

For example, in this April, 2012, study, researchers concluded that the curcuminoid extract of turmeric was able to reduce inflammation in patients who suffered from knee osteoarthritis. They published those findings in the" Indonesian Journal of Internal Medicine." In this study, they compared the effect of a curcuminoid extract to the NSAID drug diclofenac sodium. The subjects were given either 30 mg of turmeric extract (curcuminoid) three times daily or 25 mg of diclofenac sodium three times daily for four weeks. After the treatment period, do you know what they found? Both curcuminoid and diclofenac sodium were both equally capable of dramatically decreasing the secretion of the inflammatory cox-2 enzyme with nearly identical results and potency.

And, this wasn't the first human study to prove that turmeric is at least as effective as an NSAID in decreasing osteoarthritis symptoms. A 2010 study published in "The Journal of Alternative and Complementary Medicine" concluded that 2,000 mg of turmeric extract was equally as effective as 800 mg of ibuprofen in reducing symptoms of pain and inflammation.[ii] And, a 2004 study published in" Oncogene" found that curcumin (as well as resveratrol) were effective alternatives to aspirin, ibuprofen, sulindac, phenylbutazone, naproxen, indomethacin, diclofenac, dexamethasone, celecoxib, and tamoxifen in exerting anti-inflammatory and anti-proliferative activity against tumor cells.

There have been numerous studies done confirming that turmeric curcuminoids have very effective anti-inflammatory properties, so that's nothing new. What's really interesting is that this most recent study not only confirms what we already knew, but also proves the natural solution is just as effective as the NSAID drugs without causing any negative side effects. Yet NSAID drugs, like the ever popular diclofenac, have been linked to many health problems such as the following: increased cardiac mortality, miscarriages and seizures.

- **Oxaliplatin (chemotherapy drug)**: According to a 2007 study published in the International Journal of Cancer, curcumin compares favorably with oxaliplatin as an antiproliferative agent in colorectal cell lines.[viii]
- **Metformin (diabetes drug)**: A 2009 study published in Biochemistry and Biophysical Research Community revealed that curcumin might be valuable in treating diabetes because it activates AMPK (which increases glucose uptake) and suppresses gluconeogenic gene expression (which suppresses glucose production in the liver) in hepatoma cells. Plus, the researchers found that curcumin was 500 to 100,000 times (in the form known as tetrahydrocurcuminoids) more potent than metformin in activating AMPK and its downstream target acetyl-CoA carboxylase (ACC). [ix]
- **Turmeric** has also proven effective in research on drug resistant and multi-drug resistant cancers. While there are numerous substances with demonstrable efficacy against these chemotherapy-resistant and radiation-resistant cancers, curcumin is the best.

In fact, there are at least 54 studies that indicate curcumin is able to cause cell death in drug-resistant cancer growths and another 27 studies on curcumin's ability to enable the cell lines to better receive conventional treatment. [x] [xi]

- **Turmeric** is also making big waves in the world of Alzheimer's disease (AD), which is the most common type of dementia. A recent study indicates that patients with (AD) who were given less than a gram of turmeric daily over a three-month timeframe had marked improvement. According to the study, all three patients involved in this three-month venture suffered from irritability, agitation, anxiety and apathy, and two of the three battled urinary incontinence and wonderings. After taking the turmeric powder capsules, their symptoms began subsiding without any adverse repercussions. ("Effects of turmeric on Alzheimer's disease with behavioral and psychological symptoms of dementia." [iii]).

Of course, this is no surprise to those living in India . For more than 5,000 years, the Indian people have used turmeric in their food on a daily basis, which is why both rural and urban populations of India have some of the lowest occurrences of AD in the entire world. So, why is the Western World so far behind when it comes to using natural means to treat and prevent illnesses instead of treating every disease with drugs that cause adverse side effects? Well, human research on the health benefits of turmeric is lacking, even though the animal studies have been extensive. This is mainly because of a lack of funding for the needed expensive human clinical trials. Unfortunately, the handwriting is on the wall. The FDA will never give its stamp of approval on turmeric, no matter how amazing it is or how many health benefits it provides. Why? Turmeric grows wild and is in ample supply, meaning it isn't exclusive, and it has no patentability which translates into no profitability. It all comes down to the old saying, "He who owns the gold makes the rules." So, unless a private investor is willing to spend about $800 million upfront to conduct multi-phased, double-blind, randomized clinical trials, they will never happen. [xii]

With turmeric's (curcumin's) strong track record as a drug alternative or preventative weapon against many diseases, it's no wonder why so many cultures have used it as both food and medicine for thousands of years. But, now it's time that we begin implementing turmeric into our diets on purpose and with consistency—with or without an FDA stamp of approval. My advice is to use certified organic (non-irradiated) turmeric in low culinary doses every day so that you won't have to consume massive amounts in later years if a serious disease should creep into your life.

Resources:

[i] P Usharani, A A Mateen, M U R Naidu, Y S N Raju , Naval Chandra. Effect of NCB-02, atorvastatin and placebo on endothelial function, oxidative stress and inflammatory markers in patients with type 2 diabetes mellitus: a randomized, parallel-group, placebo-controlled, 8-week study. Drugs R D. 2008;9(4):243-50. PMID: 18588355

[ii] B Lal, A K Kapoor, O P Asthana, P K Agrawal, R Prasad, P Kumar, R C Srimal. Efficacy of curcumin in the management of chronic anterior uveitis. Phytother Res. 1999 Jun;13(4):318-22. PMID: 10404539

[iii] Jiayuan Sun, Weigang Guo, Yong Ben, Jinjun Jiang, Changjun Tan, Zude Xu, Xiangdong Wang, Chunxue Bai. Preventive effects of curcumin and dexamethasone on lung transplantation-associated lung injury in rats. Crit Care Med. 2008 Apr;36(4):1205-13. PMID: 18379247

[iv] J Sun, D Yang, S Li, Z Xu, X Wang, C Bai. Effects of curcumin or dexamethasone on lung ischaemia-reperfusion injury in rats. Cancer Lett. 2003 Mar 31;192(2):145-9. PMID: 18799504

[v] Jayesh Sanmukhani, Ashish Anovadiya, Chandrabhanu B Tripathi. Evaluation of antidepressant like activity of curcumin and its combination with fluoxetine and imipramine: an acute and chronic study. Acta Pol Pharm. 2011 Sep-Oct;68(5):769-75. PMID: 21928724

[vi] R Srivastava, V Puri, R C Srimal, B N Dhawan . Effect of curcumin on platelet aggregation and vascular prostacyclin synthesis. Arzneimittelforschung. 1986 Apr;36(4):715-7. PMID: 3521617

[vii] Yasunari Takada, Anjana Bhardwaj, Pravin Potdar, Bharat B Aggarwal. Nonsteroidal anti-inflammatory agents differ in their ability to suppress NF-kappaB activation, inhibition of expression of cyclooxygenase-2 and cyclin D1, and abrogation of tumor cell proliferation. Oncogene. 2004 Dec 9;23(57):9247-58. PMID: 15489888

[viii] Lynne M Howells, Anita Mitra, Margaret M Manson. Comparison of oxaliplatin- and curcumin-mediated antiproliferative effects in colorectal cell lines. Int J Cancer. 2007 Jul 1;121(1):175-83. PMID: 17330230

[ix] Teayoun Kim, Jessica Davis, Albert J Zhang, Xiaoming He, Suresh T Mathews. Curcumin activates AMPK and suppresses gluconeogenic gene expression in hepatoma cells. Biochem Biophys Res Commun. 2009 Oct 16;388(2):377-82. Epub 2009 Aug 8. PMID: 19665995

[x] GreenMedInfo.com, Curcumin Kills Drug Resistant Cancers, 54 Abstracts

[xi] GreenMedInfo.com, Curcumin Kills Multi-Drug Resistant Cancers: 27 Abstracts.

[xii] GreenMedInfo.com, Why The Law Forbids The Medicinal Use of Natural Substances Feb. 26th, 2012

44 Dangerous Drugs and their Side Effects

TEN OF THE MOST DANGEROUS DRUGS APPROVED FOR USAGE IN AMERICA

This was a very difficult chapter to write. Not because there wasn't enough material but because there is too much material. There are so many dangerous drugs that are being used globally that it is difficult for me to pick just ten. This is why this list was developed by category of treatment. not just specific drugs.

But before I start I want you to know that in some cases drugs ARE necessary. So as another reminder, please do not use this chapter to decide not to take a prescription drug. Before discontinuing any prescription drug you MUST consult with you physician who gave you the prescription. Some of these drugs have severe consequences, including death, if stopped abruptly. Do NOT stop taking a prescription drug without consulting with your physician.

If your physician is not willing to help you find available natural alternatives to prescription drugs, I strongly suggest for you to get a second or third opinion.

The side effects listed do not happen to everyone. Some of the side effects are very rare. I am not going to comment on the side effects as they are self-explanatory. To do so, would require several more books. Again, as I have urged you many times in this book do you own research. Have the pharmacist or doctor give you the list of side effects before you fill the prescription. Then you and your doctor decide if the prescription is worth the risk. Because, in many cases, the prescription can cause more harm that the condition being treated. Again, If you have any questions call your physician.

The following are the drugs chosen by me to list their side effects:

Dementia and Alzheimer's:

Severe allergic reactions (rash; hives; itching; difficulty breathing; tightness in the chest; swelling of the mouth, face, lips, or tongue); bloody or black, tarry stools; chest pain; decreased, difficult, or painful urination; fainting; fever; flu-like symptoms (for example, headache, muscle aches, tiredness); mood or mental problems (for example, depression); new or worsening breathing problems (for example, shortness of breath); seizures; severe dizziness or headache; severe or persistent heartburn or stomach pain; slow or irregular heartbeat; swelling of the hands, ankles, or feet; tremor; unusual bruising; unusual tiredness or weakness; vomit that looks like blood or coffee grounds.

Sleeping Pills:

Clumsiness or unsteadiness; confusion; mental depression ; dizziness, lightheadedness, or fainting; ; falling; fast heartbeat; hallucinations (seeing, hearing, or feeling things that are not irritability; wheezing or difficulty with breathing; clumsiness or unsteadiness (severe) dizziness (severe); double vision or other vision problems; drowsiness (severe); nausea (severe); slow heartbeat; troubled breathing; vomiting (severe); Sleepiness or unusual drowsiness; Abdominal or stomach pain; abnormal or decreased touch sensation; abnormal sensation of movement; appetite disorder; balance disorder; binge eating; bladder pain; bloated; bloody or cloudy urine; burning, crawling, itching, numbness, prickling, "pins and needles", or tingling feelings; change in hearing; chest discomfort; chills; confusion about identity, place, and time; constipation; continuing ringing or buzzing or other unexplained noise in the ears; daytime drowsiness; diarrhea; difficult, burning, or painful urination; difficulty with moving; difficulty with swallowing; discouragement; double vision or other vision problems; drugged feelings; dryness of mouth; ear drainage; ear ache; excess air or gas in the stomach or intestines; eye redness; false or unusual sense of well-being; fear; feeling of unreality; feeling sad or empty; fever; frequent bowel movements; frequent urge to urinate; full feeling; general feeling of discomfort or illness; generalized slowing of mental and physical activity; headache; hearing loss; heartburn; hives or welt itching; lack of appetite; lack of feeling or emotion; lack or loss of self-control; lack or loss of strength; longer or heavier menstrual cycle; loss of balance; loss of interest or pleasure; memory problems; mood swings; muscle aches, cramping, pain, or stiffness; nausea; nervousness; nightmares or unusual dreams; pain in the joints; passing gas; redness of the skin; redness or soreness of the throat; sense of detachment from self or body; shortness of breath or troubled breathing; skin rash; skin wrinkling; sneezing; sore throat; stress symptoms; stuffy or runny nose; swollen joints; tiredness; trouble concentrating; trouble with sleeping; vision blurred; visual depth perception altered; vomiting.

Beta Blockers:

A slow heart rate, or in scientific terms: Bradycardia; low blood pressure; Fatigue or tiredness; Cold hands and/or feet; Dizziness or headaches; Fainting or lightheadedness due to low blood pressure, or in scientific terms: Hypotension ; Minor or chronic chest pain; Asthma gets worse instead of recovering; Depression or feeling stress without any specific causes; Heart failure signs, for example: gaining weight rapidly, shortness of breath and the swelling of your hands and feet; Allergic reactions such as getting a rash with no explanation; hives, itching, swelling of your body; wheezing or having difficulty breathing or swallowing food;

If you stop taking beta blockers too quickly, there is the possibility of having a more serious problem, such as a heart attack.

There are other possibilities of using beta blockers:

High triglycerides or high level of cholesterol; Insomnia – difficulty in sleeping; experiencing the same symptoms of diabetes; Exercise intolerance due to fatigue or tiredness.

For beta blockers eye drops, the most common side effect is temporary eye discomfort.

Diabetes:

Chest pain; decreased urine output; dilated neck veins; extreme fatigue; irregular breathing; irregular heartbeat; problems with teeth; shortness of breath; swelling of the face, fingers, feet, or lower legs; tightness in the chest; trouble with breathing; weight gain; wheezing; loss of kidney function; pain or swelling in the arms or legs without an injury;

skin swelling; trouble with breathing when active; unusual bleeding or bruising; unusual tiredness or weakness; dark urine; loss of appetite; nausea or vomiting; stomach pain; unexplained, rapid weight gain; yellow eyes or ski; cough; dry mouth; flushed, dry skin; fruit-like breath odor; headache; increased hunger; increased thirst; increased urination; loss of consciousness; muscle pain or soreness; problems with your teeth; runny or stuffy nose; sore throat; stomach ache; sweating; unexplained weight loss.

Chemotheraphy:

Tamoxifen increases the chance of cancer of the uterus (womb) in some women taking it; Tamoxifen may cause blockages to form in a vein, lung, or brain; in women, tamoxifen may cause cancer or other problems of the uterus (womb); it also causes liver cancer in rats. In addition, tamoxifen has been reported to cause cataracts and other eye problems; it may also cause the following:

Anxiety; blistering, peeling, or loosening of the skin and mucous membranes; blurred vision; cataracts in the eyes or other eye problems; change in vaginal discharge; chest pain; chills; confusion; cough; dizziness; fainting; fast heartbeat; fever; hoarseness; lightheadedness; lower back or side pain; pain or feeling of pressure in the pelvis; pain or swelling in the legs; pain, redness, or swelling in your arm or leg; painful or difficult urination; rapid shallow breathing; shortness of breath or trouble with breathing; skin rash or itching over the entire body; sweating; weakness or sleepiness; wheezing; vaginal bleeding; yellow eyes or skin; bloating; constipation; darkened urine; diarrhea; difficulty with breathing; indigestion; itching; joint or muscle pain; large, hard skin blisters; large hive-like swelling on the face, eyelids, lips, tongue, throat, hands, legs, feet, and sex organs; loss of appetite; nausea; pain in the stomach or side, possibly radiating to the back; red, irritated eyes; red skin lesions, often with a purple center; sore throat; sores, ulcers or white spots in the mouth or on the lips; unusual tiredness or weakness; vomiting; Absent, missed, or irregular periods; decrease in the amount of urine; feeling of warmth; menstrual change; snoisy, rattling breathing; redness of the face, neck, arms and occasionally, upper chest; skin changes; stopping of menstrual bleeding; swelling of the fingers, hands, feet, or lower legs; troubled breathing at rest; weight gain or loss; white or brownish vaginal discharge; Abdominal or stomach cramps; black, tarry stool; sbleeding gums; blood in the urine or stools; bluish color changes in skin color; bone pain; decreased interest in sexual intercourse; discouragement; feeling sad or empty; hair loss or thinning of the hair; headache; inability to have or keep an erection; irritability; itching in the genital area; loss of interest or pleasure; loss in sexual ability, desire, drive, or performance; nausea or vomiting ; (mild)pain; pinpoint red spots on the skin; skin rash or dryness; stomach or pelvic discomfort, aching, or heaviness; swelling; trouble concentrating; trouble with sleeping; unusual bleeding or bruising; Inability to sit still.

Antidepressants:

Restlessness; skin rash, hives, or itching; ; Chills or fever; joint or muscle pain; Anxiety; suicide; thoughts of suicide; violent behavior; cold sweats; confusion; convulsions (seizures); cool pale skin; diarrhea; difficulty with concentration; drowsiness; dryness of the mouth; excessive hunger; fast or irregular heartbeat; headache; increased sweating; increased thirst; lack of energy; mood or behavior changes; overactive reflexes; purple or red spots on the skin; racing heartbeat; shakiness or unsteady walk; shivering or shaking; talking, feeling, and acting with excitement, and with activity you cannot control; trouble with breathing; unusual or incomplete body or facial movements; unusual tiredness or weakness; abdominal or stomach pain; agitation; back or leg pains; bleeding gums; blindness; blistering, peeling, or loosening of the skin; bloating; blood in the urine or stools; bloody, black, or tarry stools; blue-yellow color blindness; blurred vision; chest pain or discomfort; clay-colored stools; constipation; continuous vomiting; cough or dry cough; dark urine; decreased urine output; decreased vision; depression; difficulty with breathing; difficulty with swallowing; dizziness or lightheadedness; eye pain; fainting; fast, pounding, or irregular heartbeat or pulse; general body swelling; high fever; high or low blood pressure; hives, itching, puffiness or swelling of the eyelids or around the eyes, face, lips, or tongue; hostility; indigestion; irregular or slow heart rate; irritability; large, hive-like swelling on the face, eyelids, lips, tongue, throat, hands, legs, feet, or sex organs; light-colored stools; loss of appetite; loss of bladder control; muscle twitching; nausea; nightmares; noisy breathing; nosebleeds; pain in the ankles or knees; painful, red lumps under the skin, mostly on the legs, pains in the stomach, side, or abdomen, possibly radiating to the back; pinpoint red spots on the skin; rapid weight gain; red or irritated eyes; red skin lesions, often with a purple center; redness, tenderness, itching, burning, or peeling of the skin; severe muscle stiffness; severe sleepiness; shortness of breath; skin rash; slurred speech; sore throat; sores, ulcers, or white spots on the lips or in the mouth; stopping of heart; sudden shortness of breath or troubled breathing; sudden weakness in the arms or legs; sudden, severe chest pain; swelling of the face, ankles, or hands; swollen or painful glands; thoughts of killing oneself; tightness in the chest; tiredness; twitching, twisting, or uncontrolled repetitive movements of the tongue, lips, face, arms, or leg; unconsciousness; unpleasant breath odor; unusual bleeding or bruising; unusual drowsiness, dullness, tiredness, weakness, or feeling of sluggishness; unusually pale skin; use of extreme physical or emotional force; vomiting of blood; wheezing; yellow eyes or skin; actions that are out of control; wanting to kill someone; change in consciousness; change in near or distance vision; change in walking and balance; clumsiness or unsteadiness; confusion as to time, place, or person; decreased awareness or responsiveness; decreased interest in sexual intercourse; difficulty in focusing eyes; dizziness, faintness, or lightheadedness when getting up suddenly from a lying or sitting position; feeling of constant movement of self or surroundings; hallucinations; high or low blood pressure; holding false beliefs that cannot be changed by fact; inability to have or keep an erection; irregular heartbeat recurrent; loss in sexual ability, desire, drive, or performance; loss of bladder control; loss of consciousness; sensation of spinning; severe muscle stiffness; severe sleepiness; shakiness in the legs, arms, hands, or feet; sweating; talking, feeling, and acting with excitement; tiredness; trembling or shaking of the hands or feet; unresponsiveness; unusual excitement, nervousness, or restlessness; unusual or incomplete body or facial movements; unusually pale skin; decreased appetite; abnormal dreams; breast enlargement or pain; change in sense of taste; changes in vision; feeling of warmth or heat; flushing or redness of the skin, especially on face and neck; ;

frequent urination; hair loss; increased appetite; increased sensitivity of the skin to sunlight; menstrual pain; stomach cramps, gas, or pain; unusual secretion of milk, in females; weight loss; yawning; cracks in the skin,loss of heat from the body; painful or prolonged erections of the penis; scaly skin; swelling of the breasts or breast soreness in both females and males; unusual milk production

After you stop using this medicine, it may still produce some side effects that need attention. During this period of time, check with your doctor immediately if you notice the following side effects:

Actions that are out of control; suicidal thoughts or actions; burning, crawling, itching, numbness, prickling, "pins and needles", or tingling feeling; crying; depersonalization; dizziness; euphoria; feeling of distress; feeling that body or surroundings are turning; general feeling of discomfort or illness; paranoia; quick to react or overreact emotionally; ; rapidly changing moods; sleeplessness; sweating; vaginal bleeding.

Schedule Two Pain Killers:

Burning, crawling, itching, numbness, prickling, "pins and needles", or tingling feelings; severe addiction; blurred vision; change in the ability to see colors, especially blue or yellow; chest pain or discomfort; confusion; cough; decreased urination; dizziness, faintness, or lightheadedness when getting up suddenly from a lying or sittingposition; fainting; fast,pounding, or irregular heartbeat or pulse; headache; hives, itching, or skin rash; increased sweating; loss of appetite; nausea or vomiting; nervousness; pounding in the ears; puffiness or swelling of the eyelids or around the eyes, face, lips, or tongue; severe constipation; severe vomiting; shakiness in the legs, arms, hands, or feet; shortness of breath; slow heartbeat; sweating or chills; wheezing; Black, tarry stools; cold, clammy skin; feeling of warmth or heat; flushing or redness of the skin, especially on the face and neck; irregular, fast or slow, or shallow breathing; lightheadedness; loss of consciousness; low blood pressure or pulse; nervousness; painful urination; pale or blue lips, fingernails, or skin; pale skin; pinpoint red spots on the skin; pounding in the ears; shakiness and unsteady walk; unsteadiness, trembling, or other problems with muscle control or coordination; unusual bleeding or bruising; very slow heartbeat; constricted, pinpoint, or small pupils; decreased awareness or responsiveness; extreme drowsiness; fever; increased blood pressure; increased thirst; lower back or side pain; muscle cramps or spasms; muscle pain or stiffness; no muscle tone or movement; severe sleepiness; swelling of the face, fingers, or lower legs; weight gain; cramps; difficulty having a bowel movement; drowsiness; false or unusual sense of well-being; relaxed and calm feeling; sleepiness or unusual drowsiness; weight loss; Absent, missed, or irregular periods; agitation; bad, unusual, or unpleasant (after) taste; change in vision; depression; dry mouth; face is warm or hot to touch; floating feeling; halos around lights; heartburn or indigestion; loss in sexual ability, desire, drive, or performance; muscle stiffness or tightness; night blindness; overbright appearance of lights; problems with muscle control; redness of the skin; skin rash; sleeplessness; stomach discomfort, upset, or pain; trouble sleeping; unable to sleep; uncontrolled eye movements; abnormal dreams; change in walking and balance; change or problem with discharge of semen; clumsiness or unsteadiness; confusion as to time, place, or person; delusions; dementia; feeling of constant movement of self or surroundings; general feeling of discomfort or illness; holding false beliefs that cannot be changed by fact; memory loss; seeing, hearing, or feeling things that are not there; sensation of spinning; unusual excitement, nervousness, or restlessness; dizziness

Cholesterol Lowering Drugs:

Fainting; fast or irregular heartbeat; Bladder pain; bloody or cloudy urine; blurred vision; body aches or pain; chills; cough; dark-colored urine; difficult, burning, or painful urination; difficulty with breathing; difficulty with moving; dry mouth; ear congestion; fever; flushed, dry skin; frequent urge to urinate; fruit-like breath odor; headache; increased hunger; increased thirst; increased ; joint pain; loss of consciousness; lower back or side pain; muscle cramps, spasms, or stiffness; muscular pain, tenderness, wasting, or weakness; nasal congestion; nausea; runny nose; sneezing; sore throat; stomachache; sweating; swelling; swollen joints; troubled breathing; unexplained weight loss; unusual tiredness or weakness; vomiting; kidney failure; Blistering, peeling, or loosening of the skin; bloating; burning, crawling, itching, numbness, prickling, "pins and needles", or tingling feelings; constipation; diarrhea; difficulty with swallowing; general tiredness and weakness; hives; indigestion; itching; large, hive-like swelling on the face, eyelids, lips, tongue, throat, hands, legs, feet, or sex organs; light-colored stools; loss of appetite; pains in the stomach, side, or abdomen, possibly radiating to the back; pale skin; puffiness or swelling of the eyelids or around the eyes, face, lips, or tongue; red skin lesions, often with a purple center;red, irritated eyes; shortness of breath; skin rash; sores, ulcers, or white spots in the mouth or on the lips; tightness in the chest; troubled breathing with exertion; unusual bleeding or bruising; upper right abdominal or stomach pain; weakness in the arms, hands, legs, or feet; wheezing; yellow eyes or skin; Acid or sour stomach; belching; burning feeling in the chest or stomach; dizziness or lightheadedness; excess air or gas in the stomach or intestines; feeling of constant movement of self or surroundings; full feeling; heartburn; lack or loss of strength; pain or tenderness around the eyes and cheekbones; passing gas; sensation of spinning; skin rash, encrusted, scaly, and oozing; sleeplessness; stomach discomfort, upset, or pain; tenderness in the stomach area; trouble sleeping; unable to sleep; Being forgetful; depression; discoloration of the skin; hair loss or thinning of the hair; inability to have or keep an erection; loss in sexual ability, desire, drive, or performance; large, hive-like swelling on the face, eyelids, lips, tongue, throat, hands, legs, feet, or sex organs; light-colored stools; loss of appetite; pains in the stomach, side, or abdomen, possibly radiating to the back; pale skin; puffiness or swelling of the eyelids or around the eyes, face, lips, or tongue; red skin lesions, often with a purple center; red, irritated eyes; shortness of b; skin rash; sores, ulcers, or white spots in the mouth or on the lips; tightness in the chest; troubled breathing with exertion; unusual bleeding or bruising; upper right abdominal or stomach pain; weakness in the arms, hands, legs, or feet; wheezing; yellow eyes or skin; Acid or sour stomach; belching; burning feeling in the chest or stomach; dizziness or lightheadedness; excess air or gas in the stomach or intestines; feeling of constant movement of self or surroundings; full feeling; heartburn; lack or loss of strength; pain or tenderness around the eyes and cheekbones; passing gas; sensation of spinning; skin rash, encrusted, scaly, and oozing;sleeplessness; stomach discomfort, upset, or pain; tenderness in the stomach area; trouble sleeping; ; inability to have or keep an erection; loss in sexual ability, desire, drive, or performance.

ADHD and ADD Medications:

Fast heartbeat; Chest pain; fever; skin rash or hives; Black, tarry stools; blood in the urine or stools; changes in vision; severe addiction; withdrawal; use of other amphetamines when discontinued; use of illegal amphetamines when discontinued; convulsions; crusting, dryness, or flaking of the skin; muscle cramps; pinpoint red spots on the skin; scaling, severe redness, soreness, or swelling of the skin; uncontrolled vocal outbursts or tics (uncontrolled and repeated body movements); unusual bleeding or bruising; Confusion; delusions (false beliefs); depersonalization (feeling like surroundings are not real); depression (severe); hallucinations (seeing, hearing, or feeling things that are not there; hives or welts; numbness of the hands; painful or difficult urination; pale skin; red, irritated eyes; red, swollen, or scaly skin; severe or sudden headache; shortness of breath; sores, ulcers, or white spots on the lips or in the mouth; sudden loss of coordination or slurring of speech; unusual behavior; unusual tiredness or weakness; weight loss; yellow skin or eyes; Agitation; confusion (severe); convulsions; dryness of the mouth or mucous membranes; false sense of well-being; fast, pounding, or irregular heartbeat; flushing; hallucinations (seeing, hearing, or feeling things that are not there); headache (severe);increased sweating; large pupils; muscle twitching; sweating; trembling or shaking; vomiting; Loss of appetite; stunted growth; nervousness; sleeplessness; trouble with sleeping; unusually warm skin; Anger; dizziness; drowsiness; fear; headache; irritability; muscle aches;

nausea; nervousness; runny nose; scalp hair loss; stomach pain; talking, feeling, and acting with excitement; Abdominal pain.

NSAIDS:

Acid or sour stomach; belching; bloating; cloudy urine; decrease in amount of urine; decrease in urine output or decrease in urine-concentrating ability; diarrhea; difficulty having a bowel movement (stool); excess air or gas in stomach or intestines; full feeling; heartburn; indigestion; itching skin; pain or discomfort in chest, upper stomach, or throat; pale skin; passing gas; nausea; noisy, rattling breathing; rash with flat lesions or small raised lesions on the skin; shortness of breath; swelling of face, fingers, hands, feet, lower legs, or ankles; troubled breathing at rest; troubled breathing with exertion; unusual bleeding or bruising; unusual tiredness or weakness; vomiting; weight gain; Abdominal cramps; stomach soreness or discomfort; Agitation; back, leg, or stomach pains; bleeding gums; blistering, peeling, loosening of skin; blood in urine or stools; bloody, black, or tarry stools; blurred vision; burning feeling in chest or stomach; change in vision; chest pain; chills; clay-colored stools; coma; confusion; constipation; cough or hoarseness; dark urine; decreased urine output; depression; difficulty breathing; difficulty swallowing; dilated neck veins; dizziness; dry mouth; extreme fatigue; fast, irregular, pounding, or racing heartbeat or pulse; fever with or without chills; frequent urination; general body swelling; general feeling of tiredness or weakness; hair loss, thinning of hair; headache; hives or welts; hostility; impaired vision; increased blood pressure; increased volume of pale, dilute urine; irregular breathing; irritability; itching; joint or muscle pain; lab results that show problems with liver; lethargy; light-colored stools; loss of appetite; lower back or side pain; muscle twitching; nosebleeds; painful or difficult urination; pains in stomach, side, or abdomen, possibly radiating to the back; pinpoint red spots on skin; puffiness or swelling of the eyelids or around the eyes, face, lips, or tongue; rash; red skin lesions, often with a purple center;irritated eyes; redness of skin; seizures; severe abdominal pain, cramping, burning; severe and continuing nausea; sore throat; sores, ulcers, or white spots in mouth or on lips; stiff neck or back; stomach upset; stupor ; swollen or painful glands; tenderness in stomach area; thirst; tightness in chest; unpleasant breath odor; upper right abdominal pain; vomiting of blood; vomiting of material that looks like coffee grounds; wheezing; yellow eyes and skin; kidney failure; Continuing ringing or buzzing or other unexplained noise in ears; hearing loss; nervousness.

45 | Getting And Keeping Everyone Healthy Is My Business!

I regularly mail out Newsletters which are most informative and cover the cutting-edge knowledge of supplements. Please visit our Healthmasters. com web site to sign up for a free email delivery of the newsletters. In many cases you may find some of the information in this book being elaborated upon, along with new information, but be sure to read the newsletters as they will reinforce what has been covered in this book.

Please feel free to call us concerning any questions you may have about the topics in this book or to order supplement mentioned in this book. Our toll-free number is **800-726-1834** or **863-967-0244**. Valuable information is also on our web site: **Healthmasters.com**

It is such a blessing to get the praise reports from men and women that we have been privileged to help.

I call you blessed!

T. B.

CPSIA information can be obtained at www.ICGtesting.com
Printed in the USA
LVOW04s0522261114

415730LV00007B/59/P